P9-AQT-155

PATIENT EDUCATION

Foundations of Practice

Karyl M. Woldum
Virginia Ryan-Morrell
Marilynn C. Towson
Kathleen A. Bower
Karen Zander
New England Medical
Center Hospitals
Boston

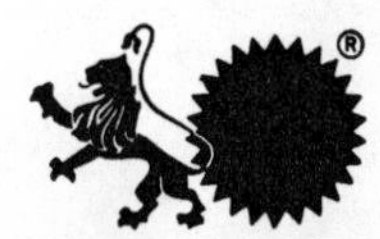

AN ASPEN PUBLICATION®
Aspen Systems Corporation
Rockville, Maryland
Royal Tunbridge Wells
1985

Library of Congress Cataloging in Publication Data
Main entry under title:

Patient education.

"An Aspen publication."
Includes bibliographies and index.
1. Patient education. 2. Nurse and patient. 3. Health education. 4. Lesson planning. I. Woldum, Karyl M. [DNLM: 1. Patient Education—nurses' instruction. W 85 P2978]
RT90.P372 1985 610.73 84-20452
ISBN: 0-89443-562-0

Publisher: John R. Marozsan
Associate Publisher: Jack W. Knowles, Jr.
Editorial Director: N. Darlene Como
Executive Managing Editor: Margot G. Raphael
Managing Editor: M. Eileen Higgins
Editorial Services: Jane Coyle
Printing and Manufacturing: Debbie Collins

Library of Congress Catalog Card Number: 84-20452
ISBN: 0-89443-562-0

Printed in the United States of America

1 2 3 4 5

Table of Contents

Preface

One component of nursing that is universal to all clinical areas of practice is patient education. At the New England Medical Center we have been interested in the dynamics that contribute to a climate that ensures patient education as a vital component of the primary nurse's role. We examined the key players (the primary nurse and the patient), their relationship, the outcomes of teaching, the teaching strategies, and finally the tools used to aid educational efforts. We found several questions related to each of these key components of the teaching and learning interaction.

- The primary nurse. Is the nurse confident in the role of an educator? Does the nurse have the skills required of a teacher?
- The patient. What are the learner's priorities and concerns? What are the factors that influence how the person learns?
- The outcomes of learning. Can compliance be predicted? Are there measures that will increase a patient's chances of implementing the treatment plan?
- The teacher and learner interaction. How is a productive relationship achieved? How is a contract based on mutual goals negotiated?
- The educational strategy. What kind of techniques are useful in achieving learning goals? What strategies are helpful to build knowledge, change attitudes, or affect behaviors?
- The teaching tool. How do you write a teaching plan or handout? How can these tools be used in conjunction with care plans?

At the New England Medical Center, we have discovered that teaching plans, handouts, and diagrams are a tremendous support to primary nurses as they assume responsibility for their patients' learning outcomes. We have also discovered that equal emphasis must be placed on developing the primary nurses' abilities, confidence, and self-image as a teacher.

This book was written to help the nurse develop in the role of patient educator. It focuses on identifying the needs of the learner according to development stages. It explores the relationship that the nurse forms with the patient and how mutual goals of learning are negotiated. Nurses teach for many reasons: to allay anxiety, help patients make informed decisions, orient patients to their environment, and, perhaps most important, change behavior. Because behavior change is an important goal of patient education, we have placed a great deal of emphasis on how nurses achieve this outcome. Finally, once the patient's learning needs and abilities have been determined, a teaching strategy must be chosen. Several strategies are explored in terms of their efficacy and application.

The editors wish to thank all those whose efforts have made this book possible—a special thanks to the members of the patient-teaching committee who worked with the contributing authors to develop the teaching plans. We also wish to acknowledge Sandra Twyon, chairman of the department of nursing, for her encouragement to complete this project and for her assistance in establishing patient teaching as a priority. Finally, this book could not have been written without Regina St. Cyr and Marie Gilarde, our secretaries, who typed the manuscript.

Chapter 1

The Nurse As Health Teacher

Karen S. Zander, RN, BSN, MSN

THE TEACHERS OF HEALTH

It has been said that every person is a hero in his or her own unique story, that "human life is the ceaseless weaving of the developmental warp of historical events with the subjective woof of our making stories about ourselves" (Rizzuto, 1978, p. 2). In this context, the patient education transaction is a meeting ground of two separate stories—that of the health care provider and that of the person seeking health-related information. The story that each of them carries and the way they build a revised version to adapt to new situations are the essence of this chapter.

People seek out health care providers when their own repertoire of skills and knowledge is not adequate for the problem at hand (Miller, 1978). For example, a mother who has tried every possible approach to her baby's unremitting rash finally enters the health care system in confusion and distress. A man who has been told that muscle spasms from playing golf are the cause of the pain down his left arm can accept that explanation until he becomes short of breath during an airplane flight.

Those people in society who have direct access to another person's physical or mental data are referred to as health care providers. Subsequently, these health care providers are the most likely to become involved in transmitting health-related information because they assume the assessment and caretaking responsibilities of the population. Thus, a person providing a health-related service, from dental hygienist to psychologist, becomes a health educator, or patient teacher. This teaching role may be passively or actively undertaken, but it is nonetheless implied as a product or byproduct of the provider-client interaction.

"Our culture is dominated by professionals who call us 'clients' and tell us of our 'needs,'" states Michael Pertschuk, chairman of the Federal Trade Commission, the agency that watches many groups claiming the title *professional* with the

Karen S. Zander is Clinical Specialist, Organizational Development in the Department of Nursing at the New England Medical Center Hospitals, Boston.

subsequent power to set standards, prices, and entry into practice requirements (Toffler, 1980, p. 50). In an age where one's health care options are plentiful it is important to study the characteristics of those whose jobs and careers are at least partially defined as conveyors of information—the formal teachers of society.

- Who becomes a teacher of health?
- What roots of identity are particular to teachers of health-related information?
- How does professional training begin to form one's attitudes, knowledge, and skills about transmitting health-related information?
- What influences the role of the professional nurse in patient teaching?
- What does expanding one's repertoire as a patient teacher entail?

Health Education: A Composite Definition

There are as many definitions of health and health education as there are care providers. Hefferin (1977) believes that the numerous definitions result from "attempts to synthesize highly complex concepts into a meaningful whole" (p. 67). Definitions have steadily evolved, perhaps related to the consumer movement and also to care providers' growing knowledge of interpersonal skills and learning theory. The 1973 President's Committee on Health Education covered the spectrum of possible definitions by stating that "health education is a process that bridges the gap between health information and health practices" (Schoemich, 1973, p. 1). Most formal definitions of health education include these characteristics:

- It is an interpersonal and, ideally, collaborative process between teacher and learner.
- It brings about knowledge, comfort, control, or other change in the learner.
- It requires knowledge and skill on the part of the teacher.

Holder (1972) views health education as a learning process aimed at changing a client's knowledge, attitudes, motivations, and behaviors through influencing the cognitive, affective, and behavioral domains of experience. Pool (1980) attends more to the therapeutic aspects of educating by distinguishing three dimensions of the health teacher's conduct:

1. supplying information with respect to the disease or the physical or social environment
2. problem counseling—paying attention to problems resulting from the disease, from being ill, or from compulsory hospitalization
3. activating patients—encouraging them to be more independent and less passive

Steckel's definition emphasizes the need to create an environment conducive to achievement of mastery and autonomy for the clients: "We [nurses] can create an environment in which the client is able to feel that there is much he can do for himself in order to maintain his health and collaborate with the provider relative to the therapeutic regimen prescribed" (1982, p. 29). She also takes a rather political stance in regard to content matter: "If we want to change our focus from disease to health, we might teach clients how to raise more questions, seek other opinions, and become generally more assertive in the health care system" (Steckel, 1982, p. 10).

The newest definition of health education includes acquisition of high-level health and maintenance of healthy behaviors. Stress-reduction, nutrition, prevention of exercise-related injuries, and fitness are considered legitimate subjects to be addressed by care providers. "Teaching-learning is important at any stage of the wellness-illness continuum but currently more emphasis is placed on teaching health promotion and early prevention" (Murray & Zentner, 1976, p. 53). This kind of definition is supported by many new groups, including Health Promotion Consultants of Cambridge, Massachusetts (Bright et al., 1979):

> Becoming healthy is an individualized process that includes emotional and attitudinal transitions along with changes in diet and lifestyle. Truly accepting responsibility for maintaining one's good health can be a challenging personal commitment. More than just following health guidelines, health maintenance is a lifelong process requiring self-awareness and personal growth. Effective health teaching therefore requires not only a thorough foundation of accurate information, but also the sensitivity and familiarity with specific techniques necessary to assist individuals through the personal steps toward a healthier lifestyle. (p. 2)

So the service of health care has, in many people's view, been linked to the service of health education. However, Hefferin (1977) gives a strong argument for the belief that "this shift in the status of patient-education—from goal to element of health care—may be more apparent than real" (p. 67):

> True, patient health education has been a provided-care service for a number of years in many settings, and there is documentation that some of these programs have been measurably effective in helping the patient toward some degree of self-care competency. For the most part, however, efforts to educate patients, their families, and the general public continue to be fragmented, haphazard, unplanned, and sporadic.

Therefore, not only do the definitions of health education vary, but also the operationalizing of those definitions varies. To get at the heart of patient teaching, we must learn in what ways health education is rooted in a care provider's skill, inspiration, and self-view.

Health Provider-Teacher Self-Views

It is important to realize that the vast majority of teachers of health are first specialists in their own fields of application and only second transmitters of health information. This "spreading" of functions is both an asset and a dilemma to health care providers-teachers and their "learners." In a global sense, the gap between provider-teacher and learner is historically outlined by Toffler (1980):

> In both capitalist and socialist industrial states, moreover, specialization was accompanied by a rising tide of professionalization. Whenever the opportunity arose for some group of specialists to monopolize esoteric knowledge and keep newcomers out of their field, professions emerged. As the Second Wave [Industrialism] advanced, the market intervened between a knowledge-holder and a client, dividing them sharply into producer and consumer. Thus, health in Second Wave societies came to be seen as a product provided by a doctor and a health-delivery bureaucracy, rather than a result of intelligent self-care (production for use) by the patient. (p. 50)

In a more immediate sense, the client seeks out a provider primarily for application of specialized knowledge (i.e., check-up, psychotherapy, emergency treatment) and secondarily for the knowledge that the professional may share. If providers do not view themselves as teachers, the client still gets "service." If providers do view themselves as teachers, the definition of that service on the market changes. The nature of that teaching service varies drastically from one provider-teacher–learner relationship to the next.

The following list shows a very simplistic differentiation between different self-views that health providers may hold:

Type of provider		*Self-view*
Global [Toffler] producer	⟶	Consumer
Service A: Provider	⟶	Client
Service B: Provider/Teacher	⟷	Client/Learner

Both Toffler's explanation and Service A represent a one-way delivery of service view of self. Service B signifies that when health providers view themselves also as teachers, the nature of the service changes because the nature of the relationship changes to a two-way exchange. The nature, effectiveness, and satisfaction levels of that exchange vary with each contact with each client.

There are three main reasons why it is extremely difficult to distinguish Service B providers from Service A providers and Service B providers from each other.

1. The roots of identity as a teacher can be quite complex.
2. Providers tend to define their standards and practice based on what they feel capable of producing. This phenomenon is probably true regarding patient teaching; i.e., if providers do not view themselves as teachers or have teaching skills, they may tend not to identify learning needs in a client.
3. The nature and outcomes of a Service B-type exchange are experienced by both participants as privately and subjectively as a physical or mental exam.

Pool (1980) claims that there is a lack of research as to what creates an inequality between patient demand for and the actual supply of health information given by doctors and nurses. He says that most of the available studies focus on the *patient's* physical or mental limitations as causative factors in the lack of communication between provider and client. To understand the health provider-teacher side of the exchange better, the authors administered a survey, the results of which are referred to throughout the text (Bower & Zander, 1983).

In this voluntary questionnaire taken by 134 health care providers, almost 90 percent stated that they were in moderate or strong agreement that "health education is one of the most important aspects of my role with patients" and "my contacts with patients and their families are incomplete if I have not included some type of teaching." Only 5 percent of the respondents disagreed with these statements, indicating a strong identity as a patient teacher across the professional disciplines represented in the sample (117 RNs, 7 MDs, 10 others). The majority of these respondents were nurses working in the intensive care units (ICUs), medical-surgical, or pediatric areas of hospitals. All but 3 of the 134 respondents described the extent of their experience as a patient educator as moderate to extensive.

Health Provider-Teacher Roots of Identity

The factors that make health providers aware of the teaching function and incorporate it into their everyday practices remain somewhat of a mystery. In the authors' survey, there was no unanimous agreement as to the definition of patient teaching, the rights and obligations of the sick role (as identified by Parsons, 1951), or the degree of confidence in the worth of the provider-teacher–client exchange. In fact, there was a quite even spread from strong agreement to strong disagreement on this statement: "Patients will make decisions about their health and adherence daily, regardless of what they may or may not know." Yet there was almost unanimous (94 percent) agreement that "my behavior during sessions with patients greatly influences their responsiveness to my teaching."

Among all the respondents, 80 percent disagreed that they "usually feel ambivalent sharing information with patients and/or their families." Most respondents (64 percent) said that they needed to know the patient's diagnosis, psychosocial background, and current life situation before they began any teaching. Persons at risk or convalescing and patients' families were ranked most satisfying to teach, while "healthy" persons ranked least satisfying. Strikingly, 87 percent of the respondents were in moderate or strong agreement with the statement, "I would feel comfortable if the teaching my patients received from me or others resulted in their seeking further opinions or becoming more assertive in the health care system."

The most personal questions of the survey focused on the providers' self-image: their own healthy behavior and attitudes and their relationship with peers. The results showed that 67 percent of the respondents agreed that "I consider myself a good model of healthy habits and attitudes," and 77 percent of the respondents agreed that their colleagues reinforced their identities as patient teachers. These results hint at trends in provider-teacher's roots but do not completely answer the question, "What makes a care provider teach?"

One's formal academic training must certainly play a part in one's identity as a patient teacher, although the degree of significance was difficult to ascertain from the survey. Only 57 percent of the respondents were in agreement that "my formal academic training adequately prepared me for patient-teaching situations I have encountered since graduation." A look at the practice of two of the largest groups of health providers—physicians and nurses—gives a confusing picture because neither group of professionals has the total market on patient teaching or has accomplished full-scale acceptance by its practitioners of the teaching role.

Physicians are traditionally seen by the public as not only care providers but also holders of information that patients need for their physical and emotional existence. Over time, that need has expanded from the proper diagnosis and recommendations to a wide variety of educational interventions. In effect, society has increased its expectations of doctors. Berish Strauch, surgeon and chairman of the division of plastic surgery at the Albert Einstein College of Medicine, commented: "The days when the doctor said 'Don't worry about it' are past. People want to know the details of what will happen and they are entitled to know" (Evans, 1983, p. 35). The need for informed consent has made an impact.

The American Medical Association's House of Delegates adopted the stance that the physician has a responsibility to provide the patient and family with education that will help them manage their own health (American Medical Association, 1975). Since that statement in 1975, there seems to be little integration of patient education philosophy and skill development at the academic level.

According to a major research study of premed students by Dr. Saul Rosenberg, a professor of medicine and radiology at the Stanford University Medical Center, too little academic attention is paid to "skills in communication, value judgments, intellectual honesty, and general education" (Hechinger, 1983, p. A3). Other physicians believe that a lack of sensitivity extends through medical school, internship, and residency: "Medicine is taught as a left-brain, scientific factual profession, without credit for feeling," stated Dr. Peter Finkelstein, who is doing research on students' responses to their medical education (Hechinger, 1983, p. A3).

Thus, one conclusion may be that training prepares the physician with the scientific background to transfer scientific information to patients but does not necessarily treat the student sensitively or teach the student how to be sensitive to patients' nonphysical needs. Weinberger asserted that medical schools could share in the government's responsibility of providing health education by teaching medical students how to educate patients (Weinberger, 1975), but it appears that there is no formal training per se.

The self-view of physicians in regard to patient education has been described as one of centralized power in which the physician, feeling totally responsible for all aspects of the patient's care, knows what is best for the patient and transmits whatever is necessary to have the patient comply. Rankin and Duffy (1983) differentiate this traditional approach to patient education from more progressive approaches in which the self-view is one of shared authority with patients, families, and other health care providers.

Yet many physicians not only see transferring some of their knowledge to clients as part of the healing role but also go one step further toward encouraging self-help and control. For instance, Richard Goldberg, a family physician at the Family Care Center of the New York Infirmary-Beekman Downtown Hospital, tells patients, "'My job is to make you as smart as you can be about what's going on with you, so you are able to take better care of yourself.' I can advise them with the best of what I have learned, but I am not a policeman. I'll give them the reasons why they should stop smoking, but I can't stop for them" (Evans, 1983, p. 35).

Similarly, Howard King, a pediatrician from Newton, Massachusetts, gives each family that enters his private practice a 44-page manual called *Kids Can Cope, and Parents Too,* a guide to the evaluation and early management of some of the common illnesses and problems of childhood. Although he states that the book "is no substitute for a frank and respectful relationship between doctor and patient," his book reflects his approach. For instance, it includes "A Glossary of Scare Terms or Words That Frighten Parents and Mean Almost Nothing Specific" (bronchitis, constipation, eczema, etc.) and a whole section encouraging families to ask what they fear are "Ridiculous Questions" (King, 1970).

Empathy for the client's situation and commitment to a physician-patient relationship that includes giving information are the signs of these physicians' approaches. They clearly see themselves as provider-teachers. Their academic training may contribute to their comfort with clients and their confidence as practitioners, but empathy and commitment are qualities, rather than skills that can be more readily taught.

Qualities are transmitted by role models in private and professional spheres of life. Thus, to learn what makes physicians move from a care provider to a care provider-teacher role may be difficult to predict or direct without an understanding of the nature of the physician's most significant role models. The possible importance of role models to a physician's teacher identity may be the factor that differentiates their "roots" from nurses who also have an identity as a patient teacher.

The nursing profession has evolved from a collective identity as general care provider and comforter (turn of the century) to that of a technician and facilitator of physician's orders (mid-1900s) to that of an autonomous profession whose phenomena of concern, theory, action, and evaluation are "the diagnosis and treatment of human responses to actual or potential health problems" (American Nurses' Association, 1980, p. 91). Thus, nursing has expanded its functional identity of health provider to health provider-teacher *by plan,* and to the extent that the definition is accepted and students and practitioners are indoctrinated, one would expect nurses to have strong identities as patient educators.

In the authors' survey of health providers in 13 Massachusetts hospitals, the significance of formal and ongoing education, personal experience as a patient or family member, and institutional and peer support was investigated. Of these, the most outstanding variable was institutional support of a teaching identity, to which 119 (88 percent) answered positively and only 9 (6 percent) answered negatively. Because almost all (91 percent) of those answering positively were nurses, a logical conclusion would be that institutional support is a significant factor in nurses' identity as teachers. One component of institutional support may well be role models. However, because nurses are employed by institutions rather than self-employed as are many MDs, the institution's sanctions and requirements may be more influential to a nurse's practice than to an MD. This hypothesis is consistent with Bosk's sociological finding that physicians do not have a corporate identity (1979).

The importance of institutional support to nurses' abilities to incorporate patient education consistently into their daily practice is described by Woldum (1980):

> It is not until nurses stop defining their roles simply as health educators and actually start implementing these roles that they realize the tremendous task they have accepted. The amount of time and expertise needed to truly educate is overwhelming. It is my belief that nurses cannot consistently implement their roles as health educators without support from their institutions. Our health institutions must not only acknowl-

> edge their commitment to patient education; they must take concrete steps to support their educators. (pp. 13–14)

An institution may support a nurse's identity as a health educator in a multitude of ways, ranging from informal, or incidental, unplanned means to highly structured mechanisms. In applying organizational development theory, the greater variety of timely strategies for encouraging or requiring certain behaviors, the more chance that those behaviors will be performed. Buhl (1979) and Nelson and Schaefer (1980) suggest a multifocused institutional approach to promoting new and complex behaviors:

- Topical. Discrete programming, which can raise consciousness toward a subject
- Programmatic. Continuous programming, which can lead toward individual behavioral change
- Structural. Systematic organizational interventions, which can produce institutional change through restructuring operations, reward systems, etc.

These three categories of planned support and reinforcement can be used to characterize current methods that nursing departments are using to foster patient teaching by nurses.

1. Topical Methods
   a. One-time seminars and workshops on patient teaching and related subjects such as contracting, working with groups, etc.
   b. Researching specific aspects of patient teaching, such as medication instruction.
2. Programmatic Methods
   a. Patient teaching and discharge planning classes in orientation programs.
   b. Patient teaching as a track of a professional development program (Woldum, Halsey, Murray, & Solovieff, 1983).

      Track A is designed to enhance the nurse's perspective of the New England Medical Center and all of its services. Activities required for participation are the development and implementation of a teaching program and membership on a standing committee.

      The teaching program should address the ongoing learning needs of a specific population of staff, patients, or families at the medical center. The programs must have clearly defined objectives, a management plan for implementation, and a stated means of evaluation. The nurse must teach the program for 9 months in order to meet the criteria for this track. Examples of teaching projects include CPR for families, instruction in the care of the newborn for families, case management for primary nurses, and games as an educational strategy for the diabetic child.

c. Programs that involve staff nurses, such as a pediatric preoperative puppet show, parents' meetings for families of hospitalized children, and health workshops for teenagers. Other programs would include cardiac rehabilitation classes, stop-smoking classes, and nurses' participation in major health screening and promotion projects such as Health Works in metropolitan Boston.

d. Discharge rounds, nursing grand rounds, and other arenas where nurses can discuss patient education.

3. Structural Methods
   a. Primary nursing, a system of care delivery by which specific nurses are held accountable for the outcomes of nursing care (one central outcome being knowledge and behavior) that their primary patients receive while on their units or clinics. The importance of primary nursing to patient teaching is discussed further in this chapter.
   b. Tools for the nurse including formal teaching plans such as offered in this text and teaching aids such as models, charts, and audiovisual supplies.
   c. Formal feedback systems, such as primary nursing supervision (a form of collegial consultation on the management of care for primary patients), incorporation of patient teaching expectations in an RN's formal evaluations, and both live and chart audits of a nurse's work.
   d. Patient and family satisfaction surveys and questionnaires.
   e. Research that includes patient teaching and is "built into" the fabric of the organization.
   f. Charging patients for health education by nurses.

The finding that institutional support structures positively influence nurse's roles as patient educators assumes that nurses already have teacher identities that require encouragement and reinforcement. Certainly a nurse's academic education provides some groundwork through socialization into the profession, whereas the patient or family needing teaching provides the stimulus to teach. The need for health education may be brought to the nurse's attention by the patient or family; by the nurse's own sensitivity, empathy, and skills in assessment, diagnosis, and intervention; or by those around the situation who recognize the need and encourage the nurse to teach. Both academic education and patient and family needs-as-stimulus must be understood to address the subject of nurses as provider-teachers.

NURSES AS TEACHERS

Nursing education has steadily incorporated the knowledge, skills, and attitudes conducive to patient teaching in its curriculum, often with the specific teaching of a disease such as diabetes as the case around which a student nurse learns the ropes. In fact, when asked to describe briefly the most satisfying patient teaching situation ever experienced, 12 of 98 RNs (roughly 12 percent) responding gave a description of diabetic-related teaching such as the following.

> Diabetic problems account, by and large, for a very significant number of comas and stuporous conditions seen in the ED (emergency department), often presenting in bizarre ways and most frequently with patients using long-acting insulin or the more potent oral hypoglycemic agents. The average diabetic patient struggles with a surprisingly inadequate knowledge of the disease process. This population is one for whom the ED nurse is in a fine position to do some really constructive teaching. Careful teaching and continued encouragement are essential to the well-being of these patients if they are to understand the disease process and care for themselves properly. (Bower & Zander, 1983)

State of the Art

The authors' survey shows that beyond teaching about specific disease entities such as diabetes and cardiac pathology, nurses derive satisfaction from teaching about upcoming surgeries and new medications. They also find great satisfaction in helping patients and families make adjustments to acute or chronic states, as shown in the following quotes:

> Being able to put a critically ill patient at ease, usually upon admission to an ICU, by constantly orienting him to what was happening and why.
>
> My most satisfying experience was preparing parents of a 4-year-old child with a chronic respiratory condition to care for him at home after 4 years of hospitalization. This family learned to competently care for their child's tracheostomy and artificial ventilation.

According to the survey, there is also great satisfaction with helping patients or their families learn how to care for themselves physically and mentally as shown in the following quotes:

> Teaching a patient with difficult wound care how to manage it at home and helping her gain her independence.
>
> . . . when dealing with patients who have had an ostomy created for whatever reason. They are so distraught but by discharge they are able to care for themselves and are able to talk about their ostomy without shame.

> I was a primary nurse for a woman with ALS (atropic lateral sclerosis) who was being discharged to home. She and her husband had a great learning need since she was being sent home with extreme weakness and on a respirator. I had to write up individualized teaching plans, do actual teaching, and then evaluate the patient's and her husband's learning.

In addition to these situations, nurses cite teaching groups of patients as most satisfying:

> Enjoyed teaching a group of diabetics about the relation between stress and blood sugar and then teaching relaxation techniques.
>
> Lead a living skills group, which was a positive experience for both myself and the patients.

In taking on the teaching role as part of the health care provider role, nurses take on a coordinating function as well:

> Teaching a mother of a new Down's baby to give digoxin. It was a very complicated social situation, which involved using social service, the cardiac nurse, intern, and other nursing staff.
>
> Assisting a family of a terminally ill patient to develop skills necessary to allow the patient to die at home (IVs, colostomy care, meds, etc.) while supporting nursing and medical staff in accepting the fact that this was the best plan for this family.

These examples demonstrate that nurses have begun to teach beyond the medical model and beyond a policing function of getting patients to "behave." In fact, teaching and nursing are united in the nurse's self-view. "Teaching is seen as one means toward the goal of nursing [independence of the client], with both the nurse and the patient assuming responsibility for movement toward that goal" (Redman, 1984, p. 2).

Certainly, teaching situations such as those quoted in the authors' survey cannot be addressed in a nurse's formal education. However, a broad enough conceptualization of the "proper" role of the nurse is taught and expected of many of today's nursing students, including

- evaluating a patient's knowledge as part of the nurse's initial assessment of the patient,
- using a health knowledge statement as a possible nursing diagnosis, and
- identifying possible behaviors of patients and their families that would indicate that, through a nurse's teaching, they have gained information, insight, control, etc.

Although nurses graduating several years ago may see patient teaching either as foreign to them (because they were never taught how to do it) or as something to do if there is enough time (because it is not an automatic part of their work), nurses graduating more recently are being exposed to and educated in a concept of their role that embodies patient teaching as central to professional nursing and nursing therapy (Mundinger, 1980, pp. 58–59):

> Nursing therapy, then, is professional because the knowledge base is unique: pathophysiology, psychology, bodily care, teaching, and counseling. Few other professionals have such repertoires of interdependent knowledge. Nursing is one of the only professions using primary physical and emotional data and intellectual and hands-on skills to identify and resolve unhealthful responses. The combination of knowledge and skill is unique. The constant interpretation of responses, close bodily care, and nurturing that allows those judgments is nursing therapy. Helping someone be the healthiest being the individual can be is the professional outcome.

Teaching As Healing

More and more, patients and their families are asking questions of their nurses. Outside a hospital they are exposed to increasing amounts of health-related information. Inside a hospital they are exposed visually to their own physical status because of modern technology showing them their uterus and fetus (as in ultrasound), their cardiac condition (as in cardiac catheterization), and their cervix (as in colposcopy). Even if they don't see their own bodies on the big screens, chances are that they will be seeing some audiovisual teaching aid or even television that is especially programmed for hospitals (Welling, 1983). They are also exposed to nurses' values about good care by the way nurses conduct their direct care delivery and the way nurses talk to them about their hospitalization. Finally, patients' awareness of health teaching is being heightened by means of questionnaires such as "Were you happy with your nursing care at Forrest General Hospital?" with 26 questions, 6 specifically addressed to patient-teaching (Ferguson & Ferguson, 1983, p. 21).

Patients want to know what is wrong, why they feel the way they do, and how to get better. They want to know how to understand, how to adapt, how to cope, how to do; some want to know how to live more "healthily." They want to be healed. Redman (1984, p. 5) contends that the goals of patient-teaching are "usually short-term and palliative rather than curative," which suggests that the self-view of the provider to become a teacher must transcend curing by moving toward healing. Although Toffler (1980) is speaking historically, his statement still holds true for health care in that there is a need for "many new kinds of specialists whose basic task is *integration*"—putting things back together in a different form (p. 61).

Whether acutely ill or extremely healthy, patients need, and if possible ask for, integration of their physical and mental experiences into an understandable and manageable condition. In other words, integration of their experiences is equivalent to healing. If nurses perceive patients' and families' questions, responses, and vast array of behaviors as a need for integration that can be facilitated, they are defining the role broadly as a teacher. If health care providers, especially nurses, do not see their healing role as teacher-integrator, patients are left angry, confused, anxious, and possibly at risk for more serious health problems.

For instance, patients in critical care units are often "unable to comprehend nurse's explanations and put them into a meaningful whole" (Roberts, 1980, p. 61), because of the acuity of their physical state, and their often-confused perception of their physical boundaries. Because they may not be able to use their cognitive skills fully, Roberts, using Piaget's theories, postulates that critically ill patients need nurses to help them integrate very basic things, such as whether parts of their bodies are intact; where their body boundaries are; what the connection is between their bodies and essential tubes, wires, and restraints; and what the sounds and people in the ICU environment have to do with them. Otherwise, "the patient's own schemata often have little resemblance to what the health care provider has attempted to communicate" (p. 61). Roberts concludes:

> The critical care nurse is the significant other and stabilizing force in the patient's threatening and dynamic environment. The nurse is the primary individual who spends the greatest amount of time with the patient. Therefore the nurse is able to accurately assess the patient's cognitive level in an attempt to help the patient assimilate and accommodate internal and external events. (p. 73)

It is not only critical care patients who require integration of multiple stimuli. Fairly healthy, knowledgeable, and motivated people do, too. The following case example is descriptive of

- the different levels of skill and style shown by various care providers,
- the influence of nonverbal activity of the health care providers,
- the fragmentation of information, and
- the lack of integration experienced by the patient as she developed her own confused story about what was happening to her.

The patient was a 35-year-old woman who just gave birth to a second child. She and her husband had attended childbirth refresher classes; although both were worried that this labor would be as long as for their first child, they were rested and ready. About one half-hour after what she was told was a normal delivery, she was eager to breast-feed the baby because she knew the importance of having her uterus contract. In fact, she had been massaging her uterus regularly as the nurses had instructed her, and it felt hard. As she sat up to feed the baby, she felt weak and lightheaded. Some of the patient teaching was in response to her questions, some was unsolicited. Chronologically, Exhibit 1–1 relates the "teaching" input that she received and her private responses to it.

What kept this case from being one of healing? Probably a combination of several uncomfortable issues did:

- The health providers themselves were confused, frightened, and possibly guilty about what was happening.
- Each provider had a somewhat different education, vocabulary, and experience level from each other and from the patient.
- Each provider had a different relationship (history, length, rapport) with the patient and her husband.
- Although certain people were in touch with the patient's own story, no *one* person had taken the responsibility of coordinating the facts or the approach to her needs.

All the health care providers probably believed that they were teaching—and they were, in the telling and information-passing aspects of teaching. What the patient feels, sees, knows, and is told, however, is a totally separate experience from what the health care providers assume or experience. Without integration of the patient's internal and external realities, the patient is never really healed. Rather, the patient is talked to—piecemeal—and becomes self-taught.

A nurse who had a self-view of a teacher-integrator-healer could have made a difference in this case. The nurse as health educator is a relatively new role definition that will not evolve further unless patient education is conceptualized as healing and all educational and work-life (structural) influences are focused within that context.

THE POTENTIATING OF THE NURSE AS HEALTH TEACHER

For the nursing profession and its members to grow as health educators, four main areas require action:

1. Education and practice must agree on the goal of potentiating nurses as health teachers.

Exhibit 1–1 Teaching Input and Responses

Time	*Input*	*Responses*
Day 1 4:45AM	Nurses put on oxygen mask, put her in trendelenberg position, started taking her blood pressure every time they entered the room.	The nurses look worried. They're taking my blood pressure a lot. I'm going to faint. The mask feels good. Normally I'd hate something on my face.
	She was informed her blood pressure was 60/20 (normal was 90/60). She asked about her pulse and was told it was 104 (normal was 60/70).	I can feel my head thumping. I'm going into shock. I can't feed the baby now—will she be all right?
	No one disturbed her husband, who was dozing in the lounge chair in the same room.	Maybe it's not serious. No one dies from childbirth anymore, do they? Will I get to talk to him before I die?
	Nurses started IV and reported that doctor gave phone order for pitocin. Baby sent to nursery.	But I've been massaging my uterus and it feels hard. The baby is getting too cold.
	Patient told husband that something was wrong. He looked surprised. She told nurses about a headache, which no one explained.	We're helpless.
6AM–11AM	After several hours and 2,000 cc IV, her blood pressure rose to 110/80. Nurses checked her prenatal records. Everytime the nurses massaged her uterus, she gushed blood. They changed her pads and sheets often. She was told she could have breakfast and that she should drink fluids.	Does the day shift know what's happening? I feel better but I don't feel safe. I'm afraid to eat solids because if I need surgery for any reason, I might aspirate. Which is worse: death by aspiration or death by hemorrhage?
11AM Transfer to postpartum unit	The floor nurse merrily said, "They hit 'high C' over in delivery about your blood pressure." "Your pads are a little brighter than normal, but no hemorrhoids!"	I feel weak. Am I still bleeding too much? What's important? Just tell me what to do and I'll do it. Did the delivery nurses tell my postpartum nurse anything specific?

Exhibit 1–1 continued

Time	*Input*	*Responses*
5PM	The doctor who delivered her visited, smiling, and when asked what happened, said: "You might have lost a little more fluid than normal. You had a lot of clots. Besides, you missed a night's sleep and were probably tired."	Is "fluid" blood? I thought clots were expected. I wasn't tired. I'd been resting 2 weeks for this delivery. Maybe he doesn't know what happened either.
10:45PM	Night nurse from delivery came to visit and said: "I was worried about you. You were in a pool of blood from your back to your knees."	Gross! Thank God I survived. I'll never be able to have another baby safely.
Day 2	When she asked the doctor why her heart was still pounding, he responded: "Your bone marrow is working overtime. We'll do a blood count."	I still feel weak, and dizzy on exertion. Don't take any more blood out! What is the connection between my bone marrow and my heart? Biology was 15 years ago! I need a cardiologist.
Day 3	The baby's pediatrician talked about how scary the postdelivery was for her, relating it to a major childhood illness he knew she had. She was able to verbalize her worries that her body was not working right.	I feel better and not so crazy. I deserve some answers.
	When the obstetrician visited, he reported "her crit is down to 25, which is low." When she offered to call her husband to bring her prenatal pills to the hospital, the doctor said he wanted her to have a bowel movement first, then risk constipation by taking iron.	What kind of crit is *too* low? I want to eat nails and lick the metal bed if it will take away the thumping and give me more energy. How can I take care of two children with no energy? What are his priorities? I'm a prisoner.
	She asked the nurses to check her pads and they said she was fine. Nurse friends told her that a hematocrit of 25 is borderline transfusion.	On, no. With my luck, something would go wrong with a transfusion. Just get me home to my iron pills.

Exhibit 1–1 continued

Time	*Input*	*Responses*
1 week Postpartum	She asked the obstetrician's partner how seriously ill she was. He explained: "It was a postpartum hemorrhage—unusual in a second pregnancy. You wouldn't have died. You would have gone to sleep while your blood was diverted to the more important organs like your heart and brain. Then you would have awakened."	I don't believe him. He's trying to placate me.
	A nurse friend told her: "A postpartum hemorrhage is anytime after the baby comes out. The muscles around your blood vessels did not contract, so clots formed to stop the bleeding." (She drew a diagram.)	That makes sense, but why me? No one did anything wrong medically. I should be thankful I have a healthy baby, and put the past behind me.
	She did not keep her 6-week checkup.	I might as well take care of myself by myself.

2. Nurses must be placed in central case management positions with patients for whom they are held accountable for outcomes of teaching, i.e., primary nursing.
3. Individual nurses must be encouraged and expected to review their own practice and set personal learning goals that will help them develop as patient teachers.
4. Nurses must become involved, initiate, and incorporate formal feedback mechanisms and research about the quality and financial consequences of the teaching role, using the data to advance nursing practice and enhance nursing's image.

The Merging of Education and Practice Expectations

If nurses believe that patients and families need clear expectations of behavior, resulting from teaching that addresses knowledge, skill, and attitudes, then the same characteristics should hold true for the nurses' own education. Yet nurses have settled for receiving less quality in their professional training and practice environments than they strive to offer patients. Clearly it is time for education and practice institutions to agree that patient education in all its forms is at the core of healing, and healing is at the core of nursing.

Hall (1983) speaks to educators' overemphasis on the assessment phase of the nursing process at the expense of minimally focusing on the other phases of the process:

> Less often do nursing educators frame courses around what practitioners do to help patients and families to change their lifeways in the direction of health. The time has come to focus on the strategies and tactics of nursing intervention with the same vigor that so successfully raised nurses' awareness of the importance of assessment in providing effective health care.

Thus, with education and practice reinforcing each other, there can be effective emphasis on the patient-teaching element of nursing intervention.

To this end, the first step is to define behavioral expectations of nurses at all levels of professional development, from entry-level graduates to highly sophisticated practitioners. Ingalls (1984) provides a useful framework for professional development by tracing the levels from introduction through innovation and discovery. By using the taxonomy of educational objectives developed under the direction of Bloom (1956) and Krathwohl (1964) and Simpson (1972) all cited in Gronlund (1978, pp. 28–33) and paralleling them with Ingalls' levels of professional development, we have a specific yet flexible grid on which to base academic curriculum, clinical performance evaluations, and career directions (see Exhibits 1–2, 1–3, and 1–4). For instance, a baccalaureate education is accountable for preparing a nurse who within a brief amount of time can function with competence in all the areas listed.

Similarly the health care setting must make it possible for that graduate to perform at the competency level. Recognizing that not every nursing service department utilizes primary nursing, and that primary nursing has many variations in practice throughout the country, the behaviors identified at the competency level may serve as a standard for all methods of care delivery. In other words, once the standards for health-teaching behaviors are agreed, various delivery models might be used to accomplish them. For instance, a professional nurse might take on an education continuity role with selected patients, or RNs, using the teaching plans in this text, might be assigned specific parts of the plans along with the physical care of their assigned patients. Any means by which patient-teaching is assessed, planned, and delivered effectively and compassionately is progress toward enhancing the self-image of nurses as teachers. Not until education and practice settings aim at the same goals will we be able to give nurses clear dictates to teach plus the background that they need.

Exhibit 1–2 Professional Development Scale of the Cognitive Domain of Patient Teaching

Patient Teaching	Cognitive
Introduction	*Knowledge* Defines patient teaching as an ongoing process between teacher and learners designed to bring about specific knowledge, skills, and attitudes in the learners.
Familiarization	*Comprehension* Gives examples of events, situations, dilemmas, etc., which necessitate some educational intervention by the nurse.
Competence	*Application* Gives examples of three actual patient cases where variables influenced the teacher and learner (i.e., stress on time, intimacy, environmental factors).
Proficiency	*Analysis* Analyzes the responses of a specific individual patient and family to teaching over a period of time as more clinical and interpersonal information is gained.
Excellence	*Synthesis* Consistently conceptualizes learning needs and their outcomes at their most basic yet workable common denominator for three specific patients and families.
Innovation/ Discovery	*Evaluation* Evaluates the advantages and disadvantages of four different teaching approaches the patient either uses or observes being used. One of the four approaches must be contracting.

The Primary Nurse As Central Provider-Teacher

To date, primary nursing is the *only* mechanism whereby individual staff nurses can be held accountable for the outcomes of nursing care (the majority of them often being outcomes of teaching) for specific patients from admission to discharge (of their unit). Clinical specialists (such as ostomy teaching nurses) should be used as resources to, not replacements for, the primary nurse. Although the primary nurse cannot possibly teach everything that patients and families need to know (due to time, access, discrepancies in expertise, etc.), the primary nurse is in the best position to know the primary patient's priority learning needs, coordinate the attainment of the various pieces of information that all the health care providers want to give, and facilitate the integration of all the input that bombards patients

Exhibit 1–3 Professional Development Scale of the Psychomotor Domain of Patient Teaching

Patient Teaching	Psychomotor
Introduction	*Perception and set* Through reviewing patient records, differentiates a learning need from (1) a behaviorally written educational objective from (2) a teaching approach.
Familiarization	*Guided response* 1. Through questioning by preceptor, accurately identifies the learning needs, deficits, and learning style of a patient and family. 2. Makes a plan to match the need with an appropriate intervention.
Competence	*Mechanism* Independently and accurately moves from a nursing assessment to a nursing diagnosis to specific aspects of at least one teaching plan for a specific patient or family.
Proficiency	*Complex overt response* Constantly revises and refines patient teaching to adjust to ongoing assessments of the patient, the health team, and own reactions to the teaching experience. Uses expressive communication techniques (i.e., nonjudgmental, open-ended questions) when teaching.
Excellence	*Adaptation* Uses creative but appropriate ways to involve at least three patients and families in their own health education (i.e., uses return demonstration, self-monitoring techniques, role play, diagrams, pictures, analogies).
Innovation/ Discovery	*Origination* Develops and conducts a patient or family health education group, game, network, audiovisual material, etc., for a minimum of eight weeks.

and families in *every* setting. Thus, the primary nurse must manage the teaching plan as strictly as the physical care plan.

Once the primary nurse is established by the institution as the central nursing care provider-teacher, the primary nurse must be established as the coordinator of the patient and family's education. This involves expanded collaboration skills so that health education can meet the requirements for effectiveness that will be delineated throughout this text. A primary nurse's ability to participate in shift

Exhibit 1–4 Professional Development Scale of the Affective Domain of Patient Teaching

Patient Teaching	Affective
Introduction	*Receiving* 1. Sees patient education as a need of patients and families regardless of the nature of their health situation. 2. States the commonalities between the nursing process and the adult learning process.
Familiarization	*Responding* Familiarizes self with at least two different texts or articles about patient teaching, healing, teaching in groups, etc. One of the references must be written by someone other than a nurse.
Competence	*Valuing* Demonstrates commitment to the purposes of patient teaching by initiating and following through with teaching assignments and documentation in the patient-teaching plan.
Proficiency	*Organization* Demonstrates the beginnings of a complex value system by actively making own and other's teaching interventions part of professional dialogue (in report, rounds, primary nurse supervision, etc.).
Excellence	*Reorganization* Sets up peer review situations for reviewing own teaching approaches for at least three different patients.
Innovation/ Discovery	*Value maturity* 1. Studies (through survey, research, etc.) assumptions, theories, or practices about patient education (i.e., compliance, usefulness of home visits, patients' perceptions of teaching, effectiveness of contracting, coordinating teaching between health providers, comparison of delivery system for patient education, etc.). 2. Formally presents findings at a class, workshop, seminar for staff.

report, multidisciplinary rounds, health care team planning meetings, and other forums during which interventions are discussed can make an enormous impact on outcomes of care. The primary nurse's self-view must be one of a patient advocate who can use a variety of power bases and allocate resources to facilitate health education.

Finally, primary nursing makes it possible for realistic and individualized outcomes of teaching to be identified and evaluated continuously. Without primary nursing, patient-teaching by nurses will continue to be a sporadic, fragmented phenomenon, subject to the vicissitudes of a work overload, the state of staff group cohesion, and the personal values of multiple individual care providers, each doing their own thing. Even with primary nursing, patient-teaching requires a major commitment from the individual nurses and their department to accomplish the role of care provider-teacher.

Expansion of One's Patient Teaching Repertoire

There is always room to grow as a patient teacher, and most of the methods are not complex. Ten steps toward taking on and identifying oneself as a provider-teacher are offered.

1. Believe in yourself and what you are doing. "The first step is to begin with ourselves by observing our own nursing practice and defining our unique contributions" (Steckel, 1982, p. 24).
2. See yourself as an extension of the client (working on the client's needs and goals) rather than an extension of the physician, nursing staff, etc. (Steckel, 1982, p. 15). Reconsider your own perception of each patient by putting yourself in that person's shoes.
3. Decrease your isolation (working different agencies, shifts, units) by setting up peer support for your teaching identity: "During discussions nurses learn from each other, teach each other new strategies, test out new ideas, and stimulate each other's thinking about nursing practice" (Steckel, 1982, p. 30).
4. See yourself as an important advocate for the patient and family but not the savior of the problem. Nurses are interdependent on systems and other providers. Learn how to advocate through the system.
5. Risk questioning your beliefs about what specific clients need and how to give it to them. Stay current with others' assessments of your clients, as well as with research about patient-teaching.
6. Let the client teach you whenever possible.
7. View every communication (both verbal and nonverbal) with a patient or family as a form of teaching, making the most of your limited time. Show patients their care plans, thus informing them about nursing's role in relation to their case.
8. Be aware of the teaching efforts of other members of the health team. Mention them, giving the patients and families the perception that everyone knows and cares about them.
9. Accept the responsibility for documenting your teaching actions and their outcomes (Steckel, 1982).
10. Experiment with one new teaching technique each year and obtain feedback on its effectiveness.

Formal Feedback To Advance Practice and Enhance Image

To date, the art and science of patient education remain elusive and subjective. Redman (1984) states that few research tools are developed specifically for patient education and even if they were, there are minimal data in patient records. However, she suggests three categories of questions that require investigation:

1. How much learning is planned and beneficial to patients?
2. Given optimal teaching conditions, how effective is patient education?
3. What learning goals or systems of treatment are obtainable?

Formal feedback in the form of clinical research to advance nursing practice and enhance nursing's image must be focused on the individual nurse-patient interaction. Tape and video recordings, process recordings, and patient interviews by a third party during and after admissions will probably tell nurses more about the nature and effectiveness of their patient teaching than any other means. To learn truly about nurses' self-views as they are translated into action, the discomfort at being studied and evaluated must be outweighed by constructive feedback that is generated by the research. Feedback from peers, audits, teachers, managers, mentors, and investigators should be given as close to the teaching events being studied as possible, and opportunities for repeated evaluations of a nurse's teaching behavior should be part of the research.

There is much to learn about the effectiveness of patient teaching by nurses. This text asks as many questions as it answers, yet all nurses who have seen the consequences of their teaching know the power and satisfaction involved. Steckel (1982) concludes, "As medicine did with the Disease Model, so too must we isolate nursing's unique contribution to the welfare of our clients and provide data to demonstrate a cause-and-effect relationship" (p. 23).

SUMMARY

It has been said that "health education is everyone's concern and no one's responsibility" (Weinberger, 1975, p. 138). It is clear, however, that

> nurses, by virtue of their numbers and amount of patient contact, have the greatest potential of any group of health professionals for exerting an impact on patient health behavior (through diagnosis and/or monitoring of adherence levels, implementing/clarifying health education and/or change strategies, enlisting the support of significant others, patient contracting, and behavior modification). (Becker & Maiman, 1980, p. 130)

With progressive education and specific institutional structures and strategies, nurses will evolve the scientific and technical body of knowledge needed for health education. Indeed, if both educational and practice institutions define patient teaching as a standard that they guarantee the public and to which they develop nurses' competencies, then nursing has already accepted the responsibility of health education.

Accountability for the outcomes of health teaching must still be addressed at the level of the individual nurse, patients, and their families because that, after all, is where the real action is. The ultimate key to a nurse's identity as a patient teacher might, in fact, reside in the privacy of the nurse–patient and family relationship, for that is where nurses perform their art.

REFERENCES

American Medical Association. (1975). *Statement on patient education*. Chicago: Author.

American Nurses' Association. (1980). *Nursing: A social policy statement*. Kansas City, MO: Author.

Becker, M., & Maiman, L. (1980). Strategies for enhancing patient compliance. *Journal of Community Health 6*(2), 113–135.

Bosk, C. (1979). *Forgive and remember: Managing medical failure*. Chicago: University of Chicago Press.

Bower, K., & Zander, K. (1983). *Attitudes and practices regarding patient-teaching/education by providers of health care*. Boston: New England Medical Center.

Bright, P., et al. (1979). *Health promotion and disease prevention—A holistic approach*. Cambridge, MA: Health Promotion Consultants.

Buhl, L.C. (1979). Professional development in the institutional setting. In *Designing teaching improvement programs*. Washington, DC: Council for the Advancement of Small Colleges.

Evans, O. (1983, August 29). Doctors, patients, and trust. *The New York Times*, p. 35.

Ferguson, G., & Ferguson, W. (1983). As patients see us. . . . *Nursing Management 14*(8), 21.

Gronlund, N. (1978). *Stating objectives for classroom instruction* (2nd ed.). New York: Macmillan Publishing Co., Inc.

Hall, J. (1983). In *Patient education: Issues, principles and guidelines*. Philadelphia: J.B. Lippincott Co.

Hechinger, F. (1983, April 19). Sensitivity found lacking in doctors' training. *The New York Times*, p. A3.

Hefferin, E.A. (1977). Patient health education: Goal or element in modern health care? *Health Values 1*(2), 67.

Holder, L. (1972). Effects of source, message, audience characteristics on health behavior compliance. *Health Science Report 87*, 343–350.

Ingalls, J. (1984). Competency model for Competency Development Corporation, Arlington, MA.

King. H. (1970). *Kids can cope, and parents too*. Newton, MA: Author.

Miller, J. (1978). *The body in question*. New York: Vintage Books.

Mundinger, M. (1980). *Autonomy in nursing*. Rockville, MD: Aspen Systems Corp.

Murray, R., & Zentner, J. (1976). Guidelines for more effective health teaching. *Nursing 76 6*(2), 44–53.

Nelson, G., & Schaefer, M. (1980). An integrated approach to developing administrators and organizations. *Journal of Nursing Administration 10*(2), 40.

Parsons, T. (1951). *The social system*. Chicago: Free Press.

Pool, J.J. (1980). Expected and actual knowledge of hospital patients. *Patient Counselling and Health Education* 2(3), 112.

Rankin, S.H., & Duffy, K.L. (1983). *Patient education: Issues, principles and guidelines*. Philadelphia: J.B. Lippincott Co.

Redman, B.K. (1984). *The process of patient education* (5th ed.). St. Louis: C.V. Mosby Co.

Rizzuto, A. (1978). *The patient as a hero*. Unpublished manuscript, p. 2.

Roberts, S. (1980, January). Piaget's theory reapplied to the critically ill. *Journal of Advanced Nursing Science*, 61–78.

Schoemich, E. (1973). Patient education in contemporary health service delivery. In *Proceedings of Workshop on Patient Education Programming* (HEW Pub. (HRA) 74–4002). Rockville, MD: Health Resources Administration.

Steckel, S.B. (1982). *Patient contracting*. Norwalk, CT: Appleton-Century-Crofts.

Toffler, A. (1980). *The third wave*. New York: Bantam Books.

Weinberger, C.W. (1975). The role of the federal government in educating the public about health. *Journal of Medical Education 5*, 138–142.

Welling, K. (1983, July 18). Mish mash: A new TV network for hospitals only. *Barrons*, p. 17.

Woldum, K. (1980). Patient education: The importance of institutional support. *Nursing Administration Quarterly*, *4*(2), 13–14.

Woldum, K., Halsey, S., Murray, M., & Solovieff, N. (1983). The professional development program: An alternative to clinical ladders. *Nursing Administration Quarterly* 7(3), 87–93.

Chapter 2

The Learner: Your Patient

Virginia Ryan-Morrell, RN

In a sense each of the patients that the nurse teaches will be a special learner. Each patient—whether a child, an adolescent, or an adult—brings a diverse background that directly affects the ability to understand and master information and skills.

How to develop the patient's teaching plan depends on multiple factors. These factors or characteristics of the learner are based on the patient's age and level of development. In this chapter we explore the characteristics of the child (preschooler and school-age), the adolescent, the adult, and the elderly patient as they pertain to teaching. Only through this careful exploration will the nurse begin to know the learner.

THE PEDIATRIC LEARNER

The experience of teaching children can provide the nurse with a unique opportunity to use a wide variety of teaching skills. The nurse will use adult learner teaching skills to teach the parents of children. Using a different set of skills, the nurse will develop a plan and approach to the preschooler, school-age child, and adolescent. In arranging to meet the learning needs of the pediatric patient, the nurse must consider the growth and development of the child and, most importantly, the child's parents. The following section discusses the characteristics of the preschooler, school-age child, and adolescent as special learners. It is important to note that on admission to the hospital, the pediatric patient regresses. This should be considered in all approaches to pediatric teaching. It should also be noted that with a sense of humor, creativity, and an endless supply of patience, the nurse will find teaching the pediatric patient quite enjoyable.

Virginia Ryan-Morrell is Associate Nurse Leader, Pediatrics, at the New England Medical Center Hospitals, Boston.

The Parent

In every pediatric teaching situation, a certain amount of time and planning is solely concerned with the child's parents. How the nurse works with parents and how they are included in teaching have a major impact on the success or failure of all teaching attempts. The parent-child relationship consists of a bond that extends beyond almost any situation. The successful pediatric patient teacher learns to utilize this bond to enhance teaching. A healthy relationship between parent and child many times is the biggest asset in the nurse's plan for teaching. The best, most direct way to the child is through the parents.

The nurse must initially explore the parents' abilities to participate in the care of the child. The following issues should be examined:

- Is the parent intellectually capable of learning the required information?
- Can the parent physically perform the required care?
- Does the parent appear to be a responsible and accountable adult?

If the answer to any of these questions is no, then it is vital that the nurse begin to explore other possible significant others in the home environment who may be able to assume some of the learning and actual care of the child.

Once it is determined that the parents will play a major role in teaching, it is important to explore other pertinent issues. The level of parental anxiety, the nature of the relationship between family members, the quality of the parent-child relationship, and the degree of parental involvement needed to implement the teaching plan should all be explored.

Level of Parental Anxiety

A sick child is a crisis in any parenting experience. At times the severity of the illness will have a direct effect on the level of parental anxiety. For some parents, however, what appears to be a fairly benign diagnosis can still produce an enormous amount of fear. Nurses should not assume what the parental anxiety level is by what they deem appropriate for the illness.

A colleague shared this experience:

> I was surprised as a new mother when my son was born with a congenital dislocated hip. To treat the problem my son had to wear a harness at home for 5 months. The care of the harness was taught to me by a nurse in about 5 minutes. I was given no written instruction, no reinforcement. Today I can honestly say that I never heard a word that nurse said to me. I was much too concerned with how uncomfortable my son looked in the harness, whether or not it would affect his walking, and if I had done something to give him this problem.

How much easier my colleague's first two weeks at home would have been had the nurse begun her teaching with a question: "What are your concerns regarding the harness, Mrs. Black?" By doing this, the nurse would have allowed the mother to share her fears, helped her cope with them, and left her much more open to the nurse's teaching.

A parent's perception or misconception of the disease can sometimes hinder teaching. There will be times when the parent's perceptions (however painful) will be accurate, and this must be dealt with in a sensitive manner.

A staff nurse was having a very difficult time getting past the initial teaching with the parents of Meg, a 3-year-old newly diagnosed with juvenile rheumatoid arthritis. When the nurse explored possible reasons for this difficulty with the parents, she discovered that they were being distracted by the fact that Meg's grandmother had arthritis and was grotesquely deformed by it. The parents' fear was that Meg would soon be equally deformed. Clearly the nurse could not unequivocally deny that Meg would never have deformed limbs, but she could certainly point out the advances made since Meg's grandmother's diagnosis and all of the measures that she would teach the parents to help avoid these deformities. Again the teaching course would have been smoother had the nurse explored these issues beforehand.

A familial disease can be an extremely painful issue for parents. The guilt associated with "giving my child this disease" is devastating and must initially be discussed and explored and then continually evaluated throughout teaching.

Nature of Family Relationships

On the initial nursing assessment of David Brown, a 4-year-old newly diagnosed diabetic, and his family, it became clear to the primary nurse that David's mother was a somewhat rigid woman who was most comfortable when in control. Mr. Brown was a more passive, reasonable man who seemed relaxed and easygoing. The primary nurse used these two different personalities to her advantage in her teaching. Although she gave both parents all the necessary information, she concentrated on teaching Mrs. Brown the exacting technique of urine testing and insulin regulation. The nurse made Mr. Brown responsible for meal planning (not necessarily cooking), using the exchange groups. Mrs. Brown's need for control was met by being held accountable for urine testing and insulin regulation (skills she performed well) and Mr. Brown was able to bring variety and creativity to David's menu by fully utilizing the exchange group list.

The Quality of the Parent-Child Relationship

In addition to assessing the relationship of the parents, the nurse must also assess the quality of the parent-child interaction. Preop cardiac surgery teaching was not progressing at all with 4-year-old Joseph, who was sullen and angry during any teaching attempts. The nurse was to discover that this was understandably so. David's parents had lied to him. Instead of telling him that he was to enter the hospital for an operation on his heart, they told him that he was going to the home of his cousin for a pajama party.

One can only imagine the rage and betrayal that Joseph felt when learning of his impending surgery. While gently exploring this with Joseph's parents, the nurse was to learn that they had lied to Joseph because they knew that he would be upset if they told him the truth.

Whether parents have the ability to be open and honest with their child and whether the child feels the freedom to ask questions and explore concerns are characteristic of the parent and child relationship that must be assessed before teaching. Most valuable teaching depends on a positive parent and child relationship.

Degree of Parental Involvement

The degree of parental involvement in patient-teaching obviously depends on the age and cognitive level of the child. For the infant, toddler, and preschooler, the parents are the main target for teaching. Although a preschooler can participate in some of the care (a 4-year-old diabetic who washes his thigh with alcohol before his mother injects the insulin), it is difficult to direct major aspects of the teaching to a child who has not yet reached the age of reason. For unless children can reason about the illness and its management, they certainly cannot be held accountable for it. Therefore parents become accountable for the learning, and principles of adult education should be utilized.

While parental involvement is still quite intense during the teaching of the school-age child, it starts to decline as the child's ability to grasp information and perform care increases. By adolescence the child generally is physically and intellectually capable of learning most aspects of the care. Unfortunately, however, the period of adolescence is one marked with tremendous emotional turmoil. The adolescent patient may not be emotionally prepared to be totally accountable for care. How the adolescent is able to cope with illness, and the adolescent's ego strength, must be carefully evaluated by the nurse before the initiation of teaching. For safety reasons, the need for parental involvement might once again become more intense.

Infants and Toddlers

As mentioned, when the patient is an infant or toddler, the main target of teaching is the parents. Keep in mind principles discussed regarding parents and also refer to characteristics of the adult learner. Being the parent of a sick child is extremely anxiety-producing, and this should be given careful consideration in planning teaching sessions.

THE PRESCHOOL LEARNER

A staff nurse entered the room of a new admission, 4-year-old Kristen, who had a ventricular septal defect and was being admitted for cardiac surgery. Kristen was a beautiful little girl with wide blue eyes and pigtails. She sat confidently on her father's knee (it was clear who held the reins in that relationship), listening to the nurse's questions. In order to evaluate Kristen's perception of her illness and to elicit information about learning needs, the nurse asked, "Kristen, can you tell me why you've come to the hospital?" Kristen looked directly at the nurse and with very sad eyes said, "It's because I have a broken heart." After brushing visions of unrequited love from her mind, the nurse realized that although Kristen could verbalize a somewhat accurate description of what was wrong, she would probably be unable to understand all of the implications of her disease.

The preschool years are marked by high energy levels along with intensive behavior. Piaget refers to the preschooler as preoperational. "The child is capable of distinguishing between the symbol or verbal label of an object and the actual object itself, an ability which forms the basis for logical thought" (Blake, Wright, & Waechter, 1970, p. 302). This period is characterized by a tremendous intellectual, emotional, and social growth.

Unlike older children and adults, who are taught with self-care the goal, preschoolers are taught with one main objective: to help decrease the anxiety that they experience in the frightening world of the hospital. It is vital that through careful exposure to teaching, the preschooler has fears and fantasies allayed and is made to feel safe (see Exhibit 2–1).

THE SCHOOL-AGE LEARNER

The school-age child offers the nurse a delightful experience in patient teaching. This bright, self-motivated child is an eager participant in learning. Unlike the preschooler, who is taught mainly for the purpose of decreasing anxiety, the school-age child is able to learn about and participate in care.

Erik Erikson states that the school-age child's task is to develop a sense of industry versus inferiority. "The major theme of this period of the psychosocical development is the child's determination to master what he is doing" (Scipien, Barnard, Chard, Howe, & Phillips, 1975, p. 163). This striving to master skills is an asset to the teaching process and should be considered in preparing to meet the child's learning needs (see Exhibit 2–2).

A Preop Puppet Show

In an effort to decrease the anxiety of preschool and school-age children who are to enter the hospital for surgery, our institution offers a preoperative puppet show

Exhibit 2–1 Patient-Teaching with the Preschooler

Characteristics	Implications for Teaching
1. Egocentric thinking. A belief that all events and situations are directly related to self. The preschooler will attach emotions (i.e., anger, hostility) to the environment (animism).	1. The nurse should give very careful explanations of why situations are as they are. There should be clear discussion of the cause and effect of events. Machines and equipment should be explained by describing what they do.
2. Magical (prelogical) thinking and fantasies. This is somewhat diminished in this age group but continues to some degree, particularly as the child regresses.	2. With each teaching session the child should be allowed to "give back" information that has been learned. This will ensure that meanings of words and procedures are clear. The nurse should make a careful choice of words. Use of nonthreatening words that will limit misconceptions is encouraged (e.g., instead of "cut open" when describing surgery, say "make an opening"). Be honest with the child. If the procedure will be painful, explain this to the child but always limit the time that the child will experience the pain; e.g., "This will hurt for a minute but then it won't hurt anymore." Give enough information but not too much. Short simple explanations are adequate. The child will generally ask for specific information. Too much information can frighten a preschooler.
3. Castration anxiety and mutilation fears. The height of this fear is at the preschool age.	3. Approach preoperative teaching carefully—gently demonstrate on a doll what will be done to the child, particularly with urological surgery. Relieve castration fears with expressions like "your penis is red and sore but it's still there." Allow the child to return demonstrations of surgery with a doll. If the situation permits, allow the child to observe the postsurgical site.

Exhibit 2–1 continued

Characteristics	Implications for Teaching
4. Development of super ego. The child has tremendous guilt feelings associated with this developmental issue.	4. Teach why the child is in the hospital in very direct terms. This will discourage equating hospitalization with being bad or naughty.
5. Working knowledge of the body along with a lengthening attention span.	5. When explaining anatomy, use simple models or diagrams. Allow the child to play with models, etc., to become more familiar with the body. Use terminology (regarding organs, etc.) that is accurate.
6. Need for play. A child learns and communicates through play.	6. Design teaching sessions so that they will be enjoyable but informative for the child. Use toys, dolls, etc., when teaching. Allow the child to be the doctor or nurse.

to all pediatric surgical candidates. The child, siblings, and parents are invited (before admission) to come and learn through the show.

Using popular TV characters (as puppets) and principles of growth and development, the show explores common fears and misconceptions of the child.

"You mean I'm not going to the hospital because I've been naughty?" one puppet asks in relief.

Through careful explanation and demonstration, equipment is made to appear a little less threatening. Members of the OR and recovery room staff are present in order that the children can meet them before surgery.

The afternoon ends with cookies and punch and a chance for the children to play with the equipment and ask questions.

Through participation in the puppet show, the preoperative child's anxiety level is lessened, making the hospital stay less traumatic for all.

THE ADOLESCENT LEARNER

The onset of adolescence marks the beginning of one of the most tumultuous periods of growth and development that the growing child experiences. The great inner turmoil brings with it mood swings, rebelliousness, anxieties, frustrations, anger, and doubts. The emotional upheaval is so pronounced that some observers have called adolescence the period of the "normal psychosis."

Exhibit 2–2 Patient-Teaching with the School-Age Child

Characteristics	Implications for Teaching
1. Mastery. The child is eager to learn and accomplish new skills.	1. After each teaching session, evaluate the child's progress through a quiz. Leave the child with information to look at between sessions. Coloring books (that teach about disease) and pamphlets (that are age-appropriate) help reinforce learning until the next session.
2. Concrete operational thought. "By the time a child reaches school age, he can understand and use certain principles of relationships between events, things, and objects" (Scipien, Barnard, Chard, Howe, & Phillips, 1975).	2. Allow the child to participate in the teaching plan. Depending on the amount of information, plan sessions that are approximately 45 minutes in length. Sessions should be no more than 2 days apart.
3. Hospital anxiety. The school-age child has fears and anxieties related to the hospital stay.	3. Discover the child's perception of the illness. Directly explain procedures, etc., before they occur.
4. Competitive behavior.	4. Use creative teaching techniques, such as games. The child will want to learn in order to win the game. School-age children enjoy winning.

Erikson (1963) states that the developmental task of the adolescent is identity versus role confusion. Adolescents struggle with issues of identity, sexual roles, and growth toward independence. One day they demand to be treated like adults and the next day require the guidance and parenting of school-age children. They reject their parents and with this rejection comes an unspeakable fear of failure. They stand on the brink of adulthood, afraid and ambivalent about taking the remaining steps toward independence. Peers are their life, offering a mechanism for testing new-found identity. And it is these struggling, searching young adults that pediatric nurses have the incredible challenge of teaching.

A primary nurse was making very slow progress in teaching 16-year-old Julie about the care of her ileal loop. Although Julie appeared to be listening to the teaching, she seldom asked questions and was frequently unable to perform return demonstrations. One evening while passing out medications, the nurse overheard Julie talking to a peer on the phone. The nurse was shocked to hear Julie say to her friend, "I don't know why they're spending so much time teaching me about this . . . thing—now that I know I can't have babies when I grow up, I don't care what happens to me."

The nurse was stunned. Where had Julie gotten the idea that she couldn't have children? She was to learn that the normal adolescent is very concerned with sexual function and that she should have addressed this issue in the early stages of her teaching. Through careful explanation of anatomy and physiology, the nurse assured Julie of her ability to bear children, and teaching (and learning) proceeded on a much smoother course.

At best, it is difficult to consider all of the adolescents' wants and needs while planning teaching. It is not easy to know the learners when the learners don't yet know themselves. A caring attitude, a genuine attempt at understanding, a knowledge of growth and development, and a sensitivity to the incredible emotional turmoil that the adolescent is experiencing are vital in preparing to meet their learning needs (see Exhibit 2–3).

THE ADULT LEARNER

With an increasing awareness of the need for patient teaching and a strong trend toward health maintenance and prevention, the nurse is left with the task of providing thorough, accurate teaching to a wide variety of adult patients. For many nurses the adult setting is the environment for all of their teaching experiences. Certainly this setting offers an exciting forum for the nurse to practice patient teaching. What makes it so exciting is the diversity of the patient population.

The nurse may one day be teaching an 80-year-old Italian woman about congestive heart failure and the next day be teaching a 26-year-old sports enthusiast about tennis elbow. The challenge to the nurse is to teach these patients in a manner to which they can relate and then retain the information. The nurse must consider socioeconomic factors, physical limitations, perceptions of illness, cognitive levels, and at-home support structures. All of this must be incorporated into the teaching plan, with care to remember that the 80-year-old woman can't see well enough to read prescriptions and the tennis player has much of his ego tied up in his athletic abilities.

What the adult patient–teacher soon learns is that "knowing your learner" is the key to successful teaching.

To begin to know the adult learner, it is helpful to explore the developmental tasks of the adult as a person in society. Robert Havighurst identifies developmental tasks of the adult as follows (1961, p. 2):

Exhibit 2–3 Patient-Teaching with the Adolescent

Characteristics	Implications for Teaching
1. Identity versus role confusion. Struggle to discover "who am I."	1. Be aware of diagnoses that may alter adolescent's identity (i.e., orthopedic injury to a football player).
2. Independence versus dependence. Child wants to be autonomous but is afraid of failure.	2. Include the adolescent in planning how learning needs will be met. Allow autonomy in scheduling teaching sessions. Be flexible with all aspects of teaching, allowing the adolescent some control. Set realistic goals with the adolescent regarding outcome. Make a contract. For safety, teach the parents information.
3. Castration anxiety. This is a resurgence of the phenomenon observed in the preschool child. By the end of adolescence this will finally be resolved.	3. Explore fears and anxieties particularly with sexually charged diagnoses. Use phrases like "other kids with your diagnosis have been concerned with this." This will allow for less distraction during teaching. Use careful, specific preop teaching. Allow observation of the surgical site. Teach the adolescent aspects of the disease that may affect sexual function.
4. Need for privacy.	4. Explore the wishes of the adolescent regarding parents' presence during teaching. May teach parents separately. Keep confidences unless it is extremely unsafe otherwise. If necessary to report them, tell adolescents and explain why.

Exhibit 2–3 continued

Characteristics	Implications for Teaching
5. Concern with body image. Adolescents are preoccupied with body image.	5. When teaching about care at home, include ways for the adolescent to maintain a comfortable body image, i.e., hair loss with chemotherapy, use of wigs. Teach about the healing times of incisions and the results that they can expect in several months.
6. Somatization. An adolescent has irrational fears for physical well-being. Frequent vague somatic complaints may often be heard.	6. Adolescent needs clear teaching regarding normal health. Explore fears regarding prognosis, etc., being honest and direct. Consistently reinforce teaching and expected outcomes of illness.
7. Increasing intelligence. An adolescent is ready to synthesize large amounts of information.	7. Use the scientific names of organs, diseases, and procedures. Plan learning sessions of 1 hour (most adolescents are used to school classes of that length). Leave literature with the adolescent to read between sessions. Be available for questions to reinforce teaching.
8. Importance of peers.	8. Assist the adolescent in teaching peers about the disease. Invite peers to the teaching sessions. Use group meetings to teach the adolescent health maintenance. Teach techniques that will help the adolescent remain "one of the guys or girls."
9. Interest in fads and experimentation.	9. Teach the adolescent implications of participating in experimentation. (Beer drinking may have serious consequences for the person with diabetes.) When possible, use fads to enhance teaching (i.e., frequent snacking is good nutrition for surgical healing).

Early adulthood (18 to 30)

- selecting a mate
- learning to live with a marriage partner
- starting a family
- rearing children
- managing a home
- getting started in an occupation
- taking on civic responsibilities
- finding a congenial social group

Middle age (30 to 55)

- achieving adult civic and social responsibility
- establishing and maintaining an economic standard of living
- assisting teenage children to become responsible, happy adults
- developing adult leisure activities
- relating to one's spouse as a person
- accepting and adjusting to the physiological changes of middle age
- adjusting to the aging process

Later maturity (55 and over)

- adjusting to decreasing physical strength and health
- adjusting to retirement and reduced income
- adjusting to the death of a spouse
- establishing an explicit affiliation with one's age group
- meeting social and civic obligations
- establishing satisfactory physical living arrangements*

The importance of the nurse's awareness of these roles of the adult cannot be underplayed. Knowing the issues that concern the adult patient as a social being is vital in establishing a comprehensive teaching plan.

Mr. Jones's primary nurse was having difficulty in gaining his cooperation during the teaching sessions. Mr. Jones seemed preoccupied and somewhat disinterested in the information that the nurse was teaching. When confronted with this, Mr. Jones admitted that he wasn't paying attention to the teaching. He was concerned about finances. Apparently his company offered no sick time benefits and this hospitalization meant that he was losing a lot of income. With two

---

*From *Developmental Tasks and Education,* 3d ed. by Robert J. Havighurst, © 1952, 1972 by Longman, Inc. Reprinted by permission of Longman, Inc., New York.

children in college, Mr. Jones was very concerned. The nurse must be prepared to assist the patient in coping with adult issues of growth and development before valuable teaching can begin. Knowles gives the nurse some valuable insight into the adult as a learner. His assumptions of andragogy (the science of teaching an adult) provide the nurse with general characteristics of the adult learner and therefore will directly influence the plan for teaching. A summary of these four concepts follows.

First, the adult's "self concept moves from one of being a dependent personality toward one of being a self directed human being" (Knowles, 1975, p. 39). Knowles suggests that as a person grows from childhood to adulthood, the perception of self changes. Adults see themselves as motivated and in control of their lives. Imagine how frustrating a hospitalization can be for adults when they lose autonomy and control as they don the patient role. Incorporating the adult patient in the planning of all the care is most important. Asking the patients to help develop a teaching plan will return some autonomy and control to them and enhance the teaching process.

Second, the adult "accumulates a growing reservoir of experience that becomes an increasing resource for learning" (Knowles, 1975, p. 39). Knowles (1975) expands this by adding that "adults have more to contribute to the learning of others, . . . adults have a richer foundation of experiences to which to relate new experiences, . . . adults have acquired a larger number of fixed habits and patterns of thought and therefore tend to be less open minded" (p. 44).

It is a wise nurse-teacher who heeds this information when teaching the adult patient. In planning the teaching for Mr. Wright, a newly diagnosed diabetic, the primary nurse was careful to elicit information from Mr. Wright about his experience with the disease. Although he had no experience with diabetes per se, he did have a child who needed injections at home. The nurse was able to extract from Mr. Wright's experience with his child's injections, when teaching him about his own insulin regimen.

Third, the adult's "readiness to learn becomes oriented increasingly to the developmental tasks of his social roles" (Knowles, 1975, p. 39). Knowles expands this by describing "teachable moments." These are times that the adult's readiness to learn is at its peak. The adult's motivation to learn is strong since learning the new information will meet a pressing need.

Mr. Johnson was recovering from a fractured femur. In attempting to meet his learning needs, the nurse had included anatomy and physiology, pathology, and some physical therapy in her teaching sessions. Mr. Johnson appeared to be a slow, somewhat unmotivated learner. When the primary nurse began teaching crutch walking, she was amazed at how quickly Mr. Johnson seemed to learn. When she commented on his motivation to learn to walk, Mr. Johnson replied, "The doctor told me that the sooner I can walk, the sooner I can go home." A successful patient teacher learns that at times it may be more conducive to the teaching plan to teach the patients what they want to know before teaching what the teachers want the patients to know.

Fourth, the adult's "time perspective changes from one of postponed application of knowledge to immediacy of application" (Knowles, 1975, p. 39). Most of the teaching that the nurse does is done with one goal in mind: to return the adult patient to a maximum state of health. What the nurse teaches in the hospital, the patient will need to utilize at home. This frequently enhances the teaching process, for the patient knows what is taught in the hospital will soon be used at home.

One more concept of Knowles that is valuable to the nurse-teacher is the concept of conditions of learning. These seem extremely relevant to the nurse-patient relationship in the hospital setting. These are all factors that have a positive effect on patient learning (Knowles, 1975):

- The learner feels a need to learn.
- The learning environment is characterized by physical comfort, mutual trust and respect, mutual helpfulness, freedom of expression, and acceptance of differences.
- The learner perceives the goals of a learning experience to be the learner's goals.
- The learner accepts a share of the responsibility for planning and operating a learning experience and therefore has a feeling of commitment toward it.
- The learner participates actively in the learning process.
- The learning process is related to and makes use of the experience of the learner.
- The learner has a sense of progress toward the goals.

THE ELDERLY LEARNER

The older patient's learning abilities, motivation, and social circumstances differ from younger patients'. Many people think that intellectual ability declines with aging; in fact, intellectual ability only changes. There are two types of intelligence: crystalline intelligence and fluid intelligence. Crystalline intelligence is the intelligence that we absorb during our lives, such as vocabulary, arithmetic, reasoning, and the ability to evaluate past experience; this increases with age. The older person learns faster than the younger person if learning requires information acquired in the past. Nurses can build on this sharpened ability by exploring past experiences, using concrete examples, and asking the elderly what they want to learn.

Fluid intelligence or the capacity to perceive relationships, reason, or think in abstract terms decreases in the elderly. Alford (1982) describes four changes in learning that result from decreased fluid intelligence:

1. slowed processing time
2. stimulus persistence
3. decreased short-term memory
4. test anxiety

Slowed Processing Time. Older patients need more time to think through and absorb new information. Therefore the nurse should break down information into small units. When teaching a list of things, explain each element on that list. For instance, the nurse explains, "Call your doctor for the following reasons: temperature over 99°, drainage from the incision, inability to take the medication, or pain." Each of these reasons should be discussed separately, accompanied by an explanation of their relationship to the patient's problem.

Stimulus Persistence. At times older people may still be thinking of the previous concept or definition as the nurse moves on to the next one. To decrease confusion, the nurse must give them time to explore each concept in its entirety and to ask questions. Again examples should be used so that the concept can be explored to its fullest.

Decreased Short-Term Memory. The elderly remember easily things that happened in the past but may have difficulty in remembering new information that was acquired yesterday. Learning can become very frustrating if patients feel that they cannot learn because they can't remember. The nurse should work with the patient to devise ways to reinforce instruction or prod the memory, for example, listing the steps of a procedure so that it can be posted for easy reference or linking the new information to a well-known past experience. If you can find a way of reinforcing old ways of doing things, it will be much more easily assimilated than introducing new behavior or knowledge. For instance, when teaching the signs and symptoms of an infection, ask the patient to recall the symptoms experienced in the past with an infected wound or cut.

Test Anxiety. Because the elderly may have trouble conceiving new relationships and remembering new information, taking tests can be very anxiety producing. The nurse must remember to stress the individual's strengths, focus on the knowledge that the patient brings to the new experience, and if tests are given, try to make them verbal exams. An elderly patient must be given a feeling of confidence.

Teaching Methods

Teaching methods should be chosen with the older person's intellectual abilities and sensory deficits in mind. Consider the print of handouts, the volume of video displays, or audiovisual aids. Ensure that the patient can hear and see you. Because the elderly may have trouble conceptualizing new ideas quickly, a slide show is usually a better teaching device than a film. A slide show can be stopped and paced more slowly to allow for greater comprehension. A film may move too fast for the older patient (Taylor, 1982).

Groups can be very helpful in teaching the elderly. Problem solving is enhanced through conversations with others who have similar problems. The elderly are cautious and may be slow to make changes in their lives. Many times a peer group can help discuss ways to adapt behavior with minimal disruption to life styles.

Written instructions, demonstrations, and return demonstrations are very useful to teach new skills. Role playing is effective in showing the real situation and allowing the patient to practice in a safe environment. Most importantly the nurse should be empathetic, willing to listen, explain, and reassure. New skills or lists should be adapted to the patient's normal routines. The nurse should act as a consultant, a person who is available to guide and support (Murray & Zentner, 1975).

The patient's family can be a valuable resource. If the family members have an understanding, caring attitude, the patient's motivation can be increased with their encouragement. Also if the family members understand the treatment plan, they can guide the elderly and assist in realistic problem solving.

To increase motivation, ask elderly patients what and how they want to learn. Because new learning is difficult, older people will brush aside anything they do not consider useful. Older persons are accustomed to being in control and doing things well or not doing them at all. The nurse must help them regain or maintain a feeling of confidence in themselves and in their ability to learn.

REFERENCES

Alford, P.M. (1982). Tips for teaching older adults. *Nursing Life 2*(1), 60–64.

Blake, Wright, & Waechter. (1970). *Nursing care of children*. Philadelphia: J.B. Lippincott Co.

Erikson, E.H. (1963). *Childhood and society*. New York: Norton and Co.

Havighurst, P. (1961). *Developmental tasks and education*. New York: David McKay Co.

Knowles, M. (1975). *The modern practice of adult education*. New York: Association Press.

Murray, R., & Zentner, J. (1975). *Nursing assessment and health promotion through the life span*. Englewood Cliffs, NJ: Prentice-Hall, Inc.

Scipien, Barnard, Chard, Howe, & Phillips. (1975). *Comprehensive pediatric nursing*. New York: McGraw-Hill Book Co.

Taylor, P. (1982). Patient teaching: Keys to more success more often. *2*(6), 25–32.

SUGGESTED READINGS

Bibace, R., & Walsh, M. Developmental stages in children's conceptions of illness. *Health Psychology 19*, 285–301.

McCormick, R.O., & Bilson-Parkevich, T. (1979). *Patient and family education and tools, techniques, and theory*. New York: John Wiley & Sons, Inc.

Murray, R., & Zentner, J. (1976). Guidelines for more effective health teaching. *Nursing 76, 6*(2), 44–53.

Petrillo, M., & Sanger, S. (1972). *Emotional care of hospitalized children*. Philadelphia: J.B. Lippincott Co.

Pontious, S. (1982). Practical Piaget: Helping children understand. *American Journal of Nursing 82*(1), 114–117.

Redman, B.K. (1972). *The process of patient teaching in nursing*. St. Louis: C.V. Mosby Co.

Salisbury, P.A., & Beer, R.S. (1982). Marketing health communications: A case study of older adults. *Health Education 13*(6), 46–49.

Tangorra, K.H. (1982). Your attitudes toward the elderly and how they affect your nursing care. *Nursing Life 2*(1), 57–59.

Whaley, L., & Wong, D. (1979). *Nursing care of infants and children*. St. Louis: C.V. Mosby Co.

Zander, K., Bower, K., Foster, S., Towson, M., Wermuth, M., & Woldum, K. (1978). *A practical manual for patient teaching*. St. Louis: C.V. Mosby.

Chapter 3

Compliance As a Patient Education Issue

Kathleen A. Bower, RN, BSN, MSN

The ultimate goals of most patient education activities are changes in patient behavior and the achievement of treatment outcomes. This implies that patient education extends beyond the process of giving patients information and includes strategies for supporting behavior changes. Before health educators can develop such strategies, however, they need to have an understanding of some of the factors that influence the health behaviors of individuals. This chapter provides a survey of many factors thought to influence health behaviors. This information is summarized in an educationally focused patient assessment form, along with additional information about the process involved in diagnosing the health education needs of individuals.

As an introduction to this topic, consider the process of learning to drive a car. If you are not a driver, select another complex skill that you have developed. Do you remember the time, effort, courage, and patience required of you and your instructor? First, new drivers must amass considerable information about how a car is operated: when one may pass another car, the rights of pedestrians, behavior at various signs, and other seemingly endless pieces of knowledge. The process does not stop when the knowledge has been transmitted from the instructor to the learner. Instead, the learner begins to develop the manual skills required to drive a car: starting the engine, braking, turning while signaling and looking in various mirrors, and shifting the gears. And the process is still not complete because the learner must now coordinate the information amassed with the newly developed skills, a complex task of integration. Most new drivers have very high anxiety levels, and some continue to be anxious drivers despite years of experience behind the wheel. They think of the power and force of cars. They consider that driving an automobile can be fatal to themselves or others. New drivers begin to realize that their safety is largely in their own hands but that others can adversely affect it.

As they gain experience, drivers learn that operating and maintaining a car is expensive and weigh those expenses against other, pressing financial considera-

---

Kathleen A. Bower is Associate Chairman in the Department of Nursing at the New England Medical Center Hospitals, Boston.

tions. Then, too, as experience accumulates, they may become more blasé about the rules of the road. A full stop at a stop sign erodes into slowing down for a quick look. Turn signals are occasionally neglected. Seat belts are not fastened for short trips. Some may begin to believe that they can go through a red light without reprisal. Others may not value their own lives or those of their fellow drivers enough to drive safely.

Therefore, learning to drive can be described as a complex process involving knowledge, skills, and the integration of both. It is also a process where the precision learned in beginning lessons may erode over time. Throughout the process, however, there is usually a very positive outlook because most individuals look forward to being able to drive. Driving becomes a convenience and perhaps ultimately a necessity.

Now consider patients for whom complex therapeutic regimens have been prescribed. They, too, must amass considerable amounts of knowledge and develop special skills. Their period of learning is also one of high anxiety and fear. Patients must integrate skills and knowledge to be able to handle the complexities of their treatment plans adequately. Frequently they must fulfill these regimens without hope of positive outcomes or without looking forward to the day when the behaviors are no longer necessary. Their prescribed therapies may be expensive and inconvenient. The various components of their prescriptions may conflict with other activities that are important to them. In fact all of the observations made about drivers, whether experienced or beginning, can apply to patients with prescribed regimens.

The behaviors that patients are asked to exhibit are often complex and demanding. Think of the number of times you may have attempted a behavior change and encountered difficulties. Many individuals attempt to lose weight or to stop smoking with marginal, if any, success. They may have inadequate systems to support them through these behavior changes. Or their attitudes, values, or beliefs do not support the desired behavior changes. Other individuals may not have the necessary knowledge to facilitate these activities.

The changes that are required of patients would be difficult for many of the practitioners prescribing them if the authors' recent survey of health practitioners is indicative of the norm. In that survey the respondents were asked to indicate their agreement or disagreement with the statement that "I believe that I could comply with the regimens prescribed for my patients 95 percent of the time." Of 129 responses, only 69 (54 percent) were in agreement. Likewise, when the statement that "I consider myself a good model of healthy habits and attitudes" was presented, 41 (32 percent) could not agree.

A logical conclusion is that the therapeutic regimens prescribed for patients involve complex behavior changes and the acquisition of knowledge. As such, the process of assisting patients fulfill the demands of their prescriptions must extend beyond the element of transmitting information.

Many factors are involved in the decisions of individuals as to whether they will comply with health recommendations. It is critical that health educators be aware of the multidimensional nature of compliance with therapeutic regimens. Becker and Maiman (1980) underscore this point when they note that "it is unlikely that any intervention attempt which ignores the multidimensionality of the problem will accomplish long-run alterations of health behaviors" (pp. 130–131).

Health care providers often intuitively "categorize" patients regarding their ability or willingness to follow instructions. A more precise approach to this aspect of patient care will be more successful than unorganized assessments. An understanding of the various elements involved will assist the health care provider in recognizing patients who may have special difficulties. In this way, more appropriate support can be made available to those patients.

To be effective, health education must help individuals acquire the knowledge that they need. However, it must also help those individuals translate the knowledge into behaviors appropriate to the health situation. As Baric (1969) notes, "An individual's decision whether to undertake a desired health action will, in the end, define a health education programme's success" (p. 25).

COMPLIANCE: THE MEANS OR THE END?

Compliance is a very thorny issue for patients and health educators. The concept of compliance is difficult to define adequately. It is equally difficult to measure compliance in daily practice. These difficulties and others make compliance a complex research topic. Health education is usually undertaken with the goal of changing the behavior of individuals. Therefore, an understanding of compliance and its complexities is important to provide a foundation for exploring health-related behaviors. This section explores the concept of compliance.

Compliance can be described in a variety of ways. In the health education context, compliance is often associated with the extent to which a person carries out a prescribed health regimen. As such it almost always involves a change in behavior—modifying, adding, deleting. In addition, some practitioners and researchers equate compliance with achievement of a treatment goal.

Others denounce the use of the term *compliance* altogether, indicating that the free will of the patient is compromised by its use or that the term has too many negative connotations. Stanitis and Ryan (1982) echo that thought in their article "Noncompliance: An Acceptable Diagnosis?" These authors discourage the use of noncompliance as a nursing diagnosis, indicating that such a "label" leads to a negative view of the patient. They write that "the fact that a client does not participate in voluntary health action should signal the need for the collection of more data or a recategorization of existing data, rather than lead the nurse to make a diagnosis of noncompliance" (p. 942).

Questions about the usefulness of the term *compliance* are difficult to answer. The answers rely heavily on the way in which compliance is defined as well as the practitioner's own values and experiences. Alternative terminology has intermittently been suggested in the literature. Terms such as *adherence, therapeutic alliance*, or *self-care* are at times offered with the implication that the connotation is less negative. Compliance, however, is usually utilized in a context that incorporates the patient's role in the decision-making process. Perhaps that is one reason that *compliance* continues to be the most universally used term in health education literature.

In the search for a description of compliance, its relationship to the achievement of a treatment goal is an important criterion for many practitioners. As noted, some practitioners equate compliance with the achievement of a treatment goal. However, that may not be advisable for a number of reasons. Cummings, Becker, Kirscht, and Levin (1982) acknowledged that measures of patient compliance that can be found in a medical record (patient weight, electrolytes, or other objective determinations, for example) have the advantage of being relatively unaffected by human judgments. They conceded, however, that those measures may not be accurate indicators of compliance since they can be affected by factors unrelated to patient compliance behavior. Obviously some patients may achieve a treatment goal without fully (or even partially) complying with a prescribed regimen. Others may faithfully fulfill each aspect of the prescription and never reach the goal. Bollin and Hart (1982) experienced this phenomenon when they examined the question "Did adhering to the therapeutic prescriptions actually result in the desired therapeutic outcome?" as part of their study of hemodialysis patients (pp. 45–46). They found that 11 of 15 patients who complied with the prescribed fluid restrictions did not achieve the treatment goal. Conversely, 1 of the 15 patients in the noncompliant group actually achieved the treatment goal.

At least two additional factors must be considered when the relationship between treatment goals and the concept of compliance is examined: the validity of the goal and the efficacy of the regimen. Clearly the regimen prescribed does not always produce the desired results. Charney (1975) emphasized the need to evaluate the efficacy of the regimen, especially drug regimens. He noted that "considering only the patient's behavior ignores the other side of the question: was it necessary to prescribe a drug at all and, if so, was the optimal medication and dosage selected?" (p. 1009). Untoward or unpredicted responses, complications or secondary problems are only a few of the possible intervening factors.

Marston (1970) summarizes the arguments against adhering to a strict relationship between compliance with a medical regimen and achievement of the treatment goals: "In most cases the actual physical condition of the patient cannot be used as a criterion of compliance, since there is rarely a simple correspondence between following a medical regimen and the subsequent state of health" (p. 313).

It is probably safest to describe compliance as a *process* whose ultimate result is ideally, but not absolutely, a positive change in health or the achievement of a treatment goal. This description also implies that compliance is not, in and of itself, a goal. It is, however, the process that may lead to accomplishment of a goal.

Elements and Characteristics of Compliance

Compliance can be further understood through a discussion of its elements and characteristics. The process of compliance involves at least three elements (Figure 3–1): (1) cognition, (2) attitude, and (3) behavior. The cognitive component of compliance refers to the individual's knowledge base about the treatment plan. Before individuals can comply with a regimen, they must know what it is they are being asked to do, how and when it is to be done, and what equipment is required. Some people have an additional, personal need to know why the treatment plan has been prescribed. As an attitude, compliance involves the individual's willingness or intention to fulfill the various components of the prescribed treatment plan. Lastly, compliance has a behavioral component. This aspect involves the actual behavior of patients as they carry out recommended treatment activities. All three components—cognition, attitude, and behavior—are intimately involved in an understanding of compliance.

Compliance has various characteristics that lend additional insight into its nature. One such characteristic is instability. The fact that a person complies with the therapeutic regimen one day does not guarantee that it will be followed the next day. Health educators have discovered this in their practice. Eighty-three percent of the authors' survey respondents could not agree with the statement "If patients initially comply with their prescriptions, they are likely to always comply." Many factors influence patient compliance and they can be activated without warning. On the other hand, it is also not safe to assume that today's noncompliant patient will never carry out a prescribed treatment activity. The patient's behavior will probably vacillate between compliance and noncompliance over time.

Figure 3–1 Three Major Aspects of Compliance

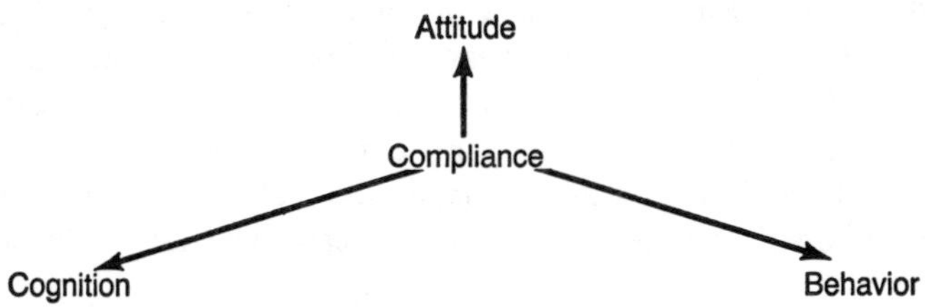

A second characteristic of compliance refers to the difficulty with which it is evaluated. Although 90 percent of the respondents to the authors' survey believed that they could tell when their patients were complying with the prescribed regimens, determining the compliance of individual patients is a complex and uncertain process. Patient self-reports, one method of gathering information about levels of compliance, are not usually considered a reliable source for a variety of reasons. Notably, patients are often reluctant or embarrassed to acknowledge that they have not carried out recommended activities. The majority (79 percent) of the health educators responding to the survey did not believe that patients are usually willing to acknowledge their noncompliance with their prescribed regimens. In fact, patients may tend to overestimate their levels of compliance.

In some situations clinical testing can be used to evaluate compliance, but even this highly objective method is easily influenced by intervening variables. Drug excretion tests have occasionally been used to determine if prescribed medications have been taken. However, if the testing is done in conjunction with scheduled clinic appointments, long-term compliance may not be measured because some patients are reminded to take their medications by the approaching visit with their health care provider. As a result, drug excretion levels are at an appropriate level when they arrive for their appointments. Unannounced home visits to determine drug excretion levels generate at least two issues: ethics and cost. Even treatment plans such as dieting for weight loss can have interference from physiological sources. The idea that compliance is difficult to measure is clearly associated with the earlier discussion about the relationship between compliance and achievement of a treatment goal. That relationship is not easily understood and is often complicated by intervening factors.

The fact that compliance is difficult to measure complicates the process of evaluating the findings of various research studies. As Marston (1970) comments:

> It is usually misleading to compare compliance rates from different studies. This is because of the wide variations in operational definitions of compliance among investigators, the lack of truly objective measures of compliance with certain recommendations such as special diets and it is the loss of precision that enters into the estimate of compliance based on several quite different medical recommendations. (p. 312)

A third characteristic associated with compliance is change. Compliance assumes a change in behavior. That change can involve the addition, deletion, or modification of a behavior or group of behaviors. Examples that describe this characteristic are easily found. One example may be drawn from the following case. Elaine Sargent is a 57-year-old woman who is about to be discharged from the hospital following treatment for an acute myocardial infarction. She was found to be hypertensive, and antihypertensive medication has been initiated. She is also 15 pounds overweight and a low-salt, reducing diet has been prescribed. Her initial assessment revealed that she smokes 1½ packs of cigarettes a day and her prescription also includes reducing or stopping smoking.

The nurse responsible for Miss Sargent's education would recognize that all three types of behavioral changes are involved in her discharge prescriptions. Her new antihypertensive medications call for an additional behavior. Her cigarette-smoking behavior is to be deleted and her dietary behavior is being modified. It is useful for the health educator to assess the types of behavior changes imposed by the prescribed treatment plan because each change creates individual problems for the patient.

Complexity is the fourth characteristic associated with compliance. Unfortunately compliance is not a matter of transmitting knowledge to patients, thus ensuring that they will proceed along the prescribed route. Experienced health educators are quite aware that there is more to the process. The relationships among the patient, the health care provider, the patient's family, the treatment regimen, and the nature of the disease process or condition are complex, and these are just some of the factors that can and will influence patient compliance. Compliance is a process that is affected by many variables and factors, some of which are not thoroughly understood.

The treatment plans prescribed are, of themselves, complex. Often patients are asked to exhibit more than one behavior in their regimens. A regimen may include a prescription for medications and exercise as well as modification in dietary patterns. Special respiratory exercises are prescribed for many patients with pulmonary diseases, for example. Follow-up appointments may be needed as well. Patients may be compliant with one aspect of their regimens but noncompliant with others.

Another factor complicating the compliance process is the reality that health issues are but one component of a broad spectrum of issues facing individuals at any given time. Gillum and Barsky (1974) observe that "each patient faces a wide array of competing demands for his time, money, energy and attention. Health care is only one of these" (p. 1564).

To summarize, compliance is a concept that is intimately associated with the patient education process. Compliance cannot be inalterably linked with the achievement of treatment goals. However, compliance can be described as a process whose ideal result is an improved or better controlled health status. There are three elements of compliance: (1) cognition, (2) attitude, and (3) behavior. Each element contributes to an understanding of compliance. An understanding of its various characteristics deepens the appreciation for compliance. Compliance is characterized by its complexity, its demand for changes in an individual's behavior, its instability, and the difficulty by which it is measured.

NONCOMPLIANCE: THE OTHER END OF THE CONTINUUM

The noncompliance of individuals absorbs vast amounts of the energy and attention of patient educators. Even though it is at the opposite end of the continuum from compliance, noncompliance is no less important or complex.

How pervasive is noncompliance? Although operational definitions of compliance vary among studies, estimates of noncompliance range from 20 to 60 percent. Some researchers cite even higher rates, particularly among those patients who are free of symptoms. Respondents to the authors' survey were equally pessimistic about their patients' compliance levels. Only 16 percent believed that most patients comply with their prescribed treatment regimens 95 percent of the time. To illustrate further, consider the research findings summarized next.

Tirrell and Hart, in their 1980 study of post-bypass graft patients, found that more than 66 percent did not comply with the heart walk aspect of their regimens. Ferguson and Bole (1979) reported that 22 percent of their arthritic patients did not comply with medication prescriptions, 60 percent did not complete their exercise programs, and 75 percent did not wear their splints as prescribed.

Bollin and Hart (1982) reported an overall compliance level of 50 percent in the hemodialysis population they studied. Becker, Drachman, and Kirscht (1972) determined, using urinary assay, that only 49.1 percent of the patients studied were compliant with their medication regimen on the fifth day of treatment for otitis media. In the same study, only 40.7 percent of the patients were compliant with follow-up appointment schedules.

A study of hemodialysis patients conducted by Cummings, Becker, Kirscht, and Levin (1982) reported that 30 percent of the patients were appropriately taking their phosphate-binding medications, 86 percent followed their diets, and 59 percent followed their fluid restrictions. Those findings were based on data available in the patients' charts. Of interest was their simultaneous finding that the patients' self-reports showed the highest compliance rates with phosphate-binding medications and the lowest compliance rates with the dietary regimen.

On the other hand, Meyers, Dolan, and Mueller (1975) reported an 80 percent compliance rate with their cystic fibrosis patients who had prescribed medication regimens. They attributed this unusually high compliance rate to the possibility that these patients and their families perceived cystic fibrosis to be very severe and that the consequences of stopping the medications were serious. In addition, the researchers felt that there were very positive patient-provider relationships.

These studies demonstrate that noncompliance is a major area of concern for health educators.

Problems Resulting from Noncompliance

There are several reasons to be concerned about noncompliance. Primarily, noncompliance may severely compromise the patient's health status. This problem increases as patients assume more and more responsibility for their health. Examples of this aspect of noncompliance can readily be found. For instance, hypertensives who do not consistently follow their regimens may develop uncontrolled hypertension, contributing to strokes and heart attacks. Adolescents who give inconsistent attention to their diabetes can develop hypo- or hyperglycemic crises, the sequelae of noncompliance.

Noncompliance can also delay or prevent recovery from a condition. As an example, teenage girls who have scoliosis must often wear bulky braces for long periods in an effort to control the curvature. Failure to do so can result in increasing malalignment, sometimes so severe that surgical correction is required.

As a result of noncompliance, the patient may be subjected to additional, and at times avoidable, procedures. As Kirscht and Rosenstock (1980) observed, "One possible ramification of nonadherence is that because a course of therapy is apparently ineffective, the therapist may try more heroic measures or shift treatment without a true evaluation of the effects of a given course of treatment" (p. 192). This places the patient at further risk for complications.

The cost of health care can be increased if noncompliance results in additional tests or prolonged hospitalization.

Health care providers find their jobs increasingly difficult in the face of noncompliance. They must try to determine why the treatment goals are not met. To make that determination, the practitioner must assess whether the problem results from noncompliance, an ineffective treatment plan, an insufficient diagnosis, a change in the underlying condition, or a combination of those possibilities. Noncompliance adds to the complexity of assessing why treatment goals are not achieved.

According to Becker and Maiman (1980), noncompliance "neutralizes the benefits of preventive or curative services" (p. 114). This is yet another reason to be concerned about noncompliance.

Noncompliance can also have a negative effect on the patient-provider relationship. Becker and Maiman (1980) note that noncompliance can negatively influence the clients' perceptions of services received. Consider the cycle that develops in the following example. The patient seeks care and is prescribed various corrective activities but does not engage in them. As a result the patient's condition does not improve, and the person becomes increasingly dissatisfied. Eventually the patient may refuse to seek further health advice.

The provider can contribute to the breakdown in the relationship with the patient. If full compliance by the patient is expected and the provider becomes frustrated or angry when it is not achieved, the patient can be rebuffed by real or perceived attitudes or criticism.

The health care providers responding to the authors' survey were asked to describe briefly, in narrative form, their feelings about or reactions to situations in which they believe their patients are not carrying out prescribed activities. Their responses appeared to be an honest reflection of the emotional and professional impact of patient noncompliance on health care providers. The overwhelming response was that of frustration. Other reactions given were a sense of failure or defeat, feelings of inadequacy, disappointment, and hopelessness as well as feeling unrewarded and upset. Anger and annoyance were also frequently mentioned. Some indicated that their time had been wasted. As one person wrote, "If patients seek medical care, then they should be willing to follow the regimen set up for them." Still others appeared to give up in that they lost interest in the patient's progress. A few indicated that they felt it necessary to relinquish the patient to another provider's care.

The reactions were strong and consistent. Many of the practitioners indicating feelings of anger and frustration noted that they tried to avoid displaying those emotions to the patient. However, there was acknowledgment that it is difficult to conceal such strong emotions. Given the intensity of the feelings reported by the respondents to the authors' survey, patient education and noncompliance are very emotional issues. Although they are understandable reactions, feelings of frustration, anger, and hopelessness can have a negative influence on the patient-provider relationship. In turn, a poor patient-provider relationship can negatively influence patient compliance. Certainly there are many opportunities for intervention along the noncompliance cycle, and the health care provider must become adept at knowing when and how to interrupt this sort of nonproductive situation.

On a more global level, noncompliance is of concern because of the effects on society at large and its health. Fuchs (1974) emphasizes this concern when he observes that "the greatest current potential for improving the health of the American people is to be found in what they do and don't do for themselves. Individual decisions about diet, exercise and smoking are of critical importance" (pp. 54–55).

Yet another reason for concern about noncompliance was raised by the respondents to the authors' survey. Those practitioners believed that it is important to identify patients who are noncompliant because 82 percent felt that they could work with the patients to increase their ability to carry out prescribed regimens.

The causes of noncompliance are not consistent or uniform from person to person. In one group, patients do not follow a treatment plan because they forget all or part of it. Sixty-two percent of the practitioners responding to the survey believe that noncompliance could be the result of patient forgetfulness. The patients who forget their treatments may be more likely to acknowledge their noncompliance than those patients who do not comply for other, complex reasons. The first group wants to comply but simply forgets to do so. A second group does not want to comply, consciously or unconsciously, for any number of reasons, including fear or conviction that the plan will not work or the diagnosis is incorrect. This group may be less willing to reveal their noncompliance. The first group (the forgetters) are likely to be responsive to supportive strategies designed to improve their compliance. The second group, however, may not respond as fully or as rapidly to such strategies (Ozuna, 1981).

The task of identifying noncompliant patients is a difficult and complex one. Some clinicians suggest that a place to begin is simply to ask the patient, in a positive way, if the prescribed treatments are being carried out. This process may help identify some compliance issues. Patients who acknowledge that they are not fulfilling their treatment programs are probably accurately portraying their situations. As Ozuna (1981) observes, "A person is unlikely to say he's not compliant when he is" (p. 4). On the other hand, evaluating patients who say that they are compliant is much more difficult because they may or may not be revealing problems with adherence to the therapeutic regimen.

Although compliance and noncompliance have been discussed as separate entities, they are really two ends of a continuum. It is a continuum with many points, and patients are probably not fixed at one point for any length of time. Rather, they move from one point to another as their situations and their perceptions change. The causes underlying noncompliance are varied and difficult to pinpoint. As Blackwell (1978) observed, "Poor compliance is the outcome of a complex interaction between the patient, physician, disease process, therapeutic regimen and the milieu" (p. 46). Therefore, it is helpful to patient educators to have an understanding of some of the factors influencing patient compliance with therapeutic regimens.

Effect of Knowledge

The following question reflects the complexity surrounding the relationship between patient compliance and knowledge. Select one answer to the multiple-choice question below that you believe accurately reflects the relationship between knowledge and compliance:

a. Patient knowledge is a major factor in patient compliance.
b. Patient knowledge does not "cause" patient compliance.
c. Both of the above statements are true.
d. Neither of the above statements is true.

The correct answer to the question is probably *c*, i.e., that patient knowledge is a major factor in patient compliance but it does not *cause* patient compliance.

A belief held by some practitioners asserts that if patients understand what they are to do, they will comply with the recommendations. Those who profess that belief assume a direct relationship between knowledge and compliance. Further, that assumption underlies the practitioner's approach to patient teaching with the result that a large percentage of teaching time is spent providing explanations, information, and directions. Is the underlying assumption a valid one? Is there a consistent, direct relationship between patient knowledge and subsequent compliance? Probably there is not.

Although patients must have knowledge about what activities they have been asked to undertake, patient knowledge has an uncertain effect on compliance. Feelings and research findings about this area are diverse. Redman (1978) observes that "patient education by itself will never solve the compliance problem because lack of patient knowledge and skill are only part of the problem. A better goal (for patient education) might be intelligent compliance, which allows and requires patient decision making within parameters" (p. 1363).

The literature is conflictive on the subject of the effects of knowledge on compliance. Blackwell (1973) espouses the belief that most compliance-related problems result from faulty patient comprehension regarding the illness, the need for treatment, and the likely consequences of both. Becker and Maiman (1980) have also commented that the patient's lack of knowledge about the prescribed regimen is a major factor in noncompliance.

Ninety percent of the practitioners responding to the authors' survey felt that if patients are noncompliant, it may be because they do not have enough knowledge to be able to comply. Only 35 percent, however, believed that "patient teaching is 95 percent a matter of explaining what needs to be done to or for the patient." Instead, they indicated that patient teaching is 95 percent a process of creating an environment in which patients feel that there are specific things they can do for themselves to maintain or return to their optimal level of health as they collaborate with health care providers. Eighty percent also mentioned that patient education must include a periodic assessment of the patient's knowledge and a regular evaluation of whether the treatment regimen is being followed.

Not all the literature supports a positive relationship between knowledge and compliance. For example, Marston (1970) writes that "knowledge per se about the illness and its treatment does not necessarily lead to compliance, although several investigators have reported such an association" (p. 318). In addition, Gutmann, Meyer, Leventhal, Gutmann, and Jackson (1979) concluded that knowledge alone is insufficient to ensure adherence to recommended treatment plans.

In general, research studies support the belief that knowledge is not the sole factor in compliance. The studies summarized next are indicative of the usual findings regarding the influence of knowledge on compliance.

A study by Cummings and his colleagues (1982) demonstrated the varying effect of knowledge on compliance. They found that knowledge about the hemodialysis regimen was significantly related to phosphorus levels but not to self-reports of phosphate-binding medication compliance. Knowledge about the purpose of the treatments was unrelated to patient reports as well as chart measures of compliance with dietary and fluid limits. Knowledge about the types of foods permitted in the regimen was not related to dietary compliance.

Hulka and her colleagues (1976) found that their group of patients were relatively knowledgeable about the medications for congestive heart failure and diabetes. Errors of commission and scheduling were higher among patients who had poor knowledge about the prescribed medications. Errors of omission were not associated with knowledge levels.

In a study of hypertensives, Gutmann et al. (1979) found that 88 percent of their study population knew the names of the prescribed drugs, 94 percent knew the medication administration schedule, and 92 percent could list two or more risks of high blood pressure. Despite the objective knowledge that these patients possessed, only 35 percent reported strict adherence to their prescribed medications.

Conversely, Vertinsky, Yang, MacLeod, and Hardwick (1976) found that increased knowledge led to increased compliance with a Tay-Sachs screening program. In a different light, Kirscht and Rosenstock (1977) found that the knowledge level of the hypertensives whom they studied was low. In fact, a number of patients were not aware of why they were being treated or why their medications had been prescribed. This group of patients showed substantially lower adherence levels with their medication regimens.

Likewise, Becker, Drachman, and Kirscht (1974), in a study of children with otitis media, found that the mothers' knowledge about how often the antibiotic was to be given was significantly ($p < .05$) correlated with compliance in administering antibiotics.

The relationship between compliance and patient knowledge is perhaps summarized best by Bollin and Hart (1982), who observed that "while knowledge does not presume compliance, it must be present for compliance to occur" (p. 43). Although seemingly contradictory, their observation does reflect the findings of these research studies. The nature of this relationship is an important one for health educators to understand and consider when developing educational strategies for their patients.

Knowledge may influence behaviors other than compliance. For example, one study found support for a relationship between knowledge and patient acceptance of medical care. Knowledge may also be a factor in continuance of care after initial contacts (Tagliacozzo & Ima, 1970).

Patients vary in what they learn. Some learn about the diagnosis but experience difficulty in retaining information about the related therapy. Others may be knowledgeable about symptoms but unable to learn about complications. In addition, knowledge about one content area does not necessarily transfer to influence compliance in other areas according to the findings of Tirrell and Hart (1980).

Clearly, knowledge has a variable influence on compliance. It is indeed frustrating to realize that if patients *do not* know the components of prescribed regimens, they *cannot* comply; but if they are knowledgeable about their regimens, they *may or may not* comply. Tirrell and Hart (1980) describe this phenomenon when they observe as part of their study that "knowledge seemed to be operating as an enabling factor in compliance but no significant relationship was found between knowledge and compliance'' (p. 492). Knowledge is not the only factor influencing compliance. Patient compliance also depends on the circumstances in which the information is received as well as on a number of other factors. Those other factors are explored in the following sections.

EFFECT OF DEMOGRAPHIC FACTORS

The effect of demographic variables on patient compliance has been studied extensively. Those demographic variables include age, sex, socioeconomic status, education, religion, and race. The results of those studies are quite varied. Some researchers report specific positive or negative correlations for one or more of the demographic factors. For example, Falvo, Woehlke, and Deichmann (1980) found that older patients had better compliance than younger patients, but no other demographic variables predicted compliance. Likewise, Nelson, Stason, Neutra, and Solomon (1980) found that a greater percentage of males were noncompliant, but other variables (such as age, education, and socioeconomic status) were not associated with compliance. On the other hand, Hulka, Cassell, Kupper, and Burdette (1976) were also unable to demonstrate a relationship between demographic variables (age, sex, marital status, education, current activity, number of people in the household, or social class) and compliance with medication regimens. Becker, Drachman, and Kirscht (1974) found that the mother's level of formal education was significantly related only to the cognitive or learnable aspects of compliance. These conflicting or nonsignificant findings are typical of most other studies involving the effects of demographic variables on patient compliance.

Health educators seem to believe that some demographic factors influence patient compliance. Those responding to the authors' survey were asked if they believed that various demographic factors strongly and consistently influence compliance. Their responses are displayed in Table 3–1.

Table 3–1 Positive Responses of Practitioners Regarding the Influence of Demographic Variables on Compliance

Variable	%
Education	76
Socioeconomic status	72
Age	68
Sex	32
Marital status	32
Religion	28
Race	23

It seems safe to assume, however, that demographic factors do not independently predict or explain compliance. In fact, Kirilloff (1981) notes that "such characteristics appear to influence compliance only when they facilitate adaptation to the particular restriction required" (p. 16). As an example, she hypothesized that dietary restrictions necessitated by a hemodialysis program may be easier for women than for men because women adjust their food preparations and preferences more easily. It has already been noted that Becker, Drachman, and Kirscht (1974) observed that the mother's level of formal education was significantly related only to the learnable aspects of compliance.

If demographic factors alone do not predict or explain compliance rates, additional factors must be examined.

RELATIONSHIP WITH THE PROVIDER

Another of the many psychosocial factors associated with compliance is the relationship between the patient and the health care provider. This factor appears extremely significant in a patient's decision to comply with the proposed regimen. There was concurrence with this proposed relationship from the respondents to the authors' survey. Seventy-four percent felt that if patients do not comply with their therapeutic regimens, it may be because they do not have a helpful relationship with a health care provider. Rosenstock and Kirscht (1980) assert that "it is known that the quality of the encounter between the patient and the provider will modify patient behavior" (p. 165). There are several factors, both positive and negative, that appear to affect patient compliance in this area.

The negative factors can be summarized into two basic categories: (1) incongruent expectations and interests and (2) dissatisfaction with the patient-provider encounter or relationship. To elaborate, the expectations held by the patient and the health care provider concerning their interaction may be in conflict. Indeed, Davis (1966) suggests that "between a doctor and a patient . . . the expectations that each has for the other are rarely congruent" (p. 1037). For example, the patient might expect to be given medication that will provide immediate relief for his cervical pain. The physician, while recognizing the need for pain medication, may focus on a regimen that requires faithful exercise and traction over at least a month's period of time. There is a significant possibility of conflict in this situation. In an extreme case, the patient may become frustrated or dissatisfied with the outcome of the visit and choose not to pursue treatment.

A conflict in the perceived needs of the patient and the interests of the health care provider may also contribute to the patient's dissatisfaction and ultimately to patient noncompliance. The health care provider may be primarily concerned with the underlying process while the patient focuses on symptom relief and a return to normal functioning. In this situation, patient frustration and dissatisfaction are an almost certain outcome.

The issue of control is key in many patient-provider relationships. Usually health care providers have greater control in the situation than does the patient. This imbalance in control is the result of a variety of variables. The provider has more specialized knowledge and skills than the patient does. Then, too, differences in socioeconomic status often contribute to the imbalance. A struggle can erupt when patients attempt to equalize control in the situation. If the practitioner does not recognize this and empathetically deal with the issue, the relationship can be negatively affected.

Interestingly, a favorable outcome from treatment is not necessarily a requirement for the patient to have a positive regard for the practitioner. For instance, in their study, Wooley, Kane, Hughes, and Wright (1978) found that 65 percent of the patients who failed to regain their usual functional status after an acute illness indicated that they were satisfied with the outcome.

Yet another potential for conflict centers around interpreting the patient's symptoms. The patient, pursuing treatment for recurrent dizziness, may be quite confused when the nurse practitioner persists in examining the patient's ears. Unless the patient's confusion is resolved, the person may continue to feel that the health care provider has not attended to the "real" problem. Lack of compliance with resulting recommendations or withdrawal from care is a likely consequence.

Patients carefully evaluate what problems are to be presented to the care provider. Part of that evaluation rests on their estimation of whether the provider can offer effective interventions. The patient's relationships with the provider also play a part. This was evident in a conversation between a patient in his mid- to late 60s and a nurse. The two obviously had a longstanding relationship as the patient enthusiastically called the nurse over when he saw her pass by the clinical waiting room. In the course of their conversation the following information emerged.

PATIENT: I don't hear so good now.

NURSE: Is that new?

PATIENT: Not really. It's been a problem over the past year.

NURSE: Have you said anything to Dr. Smythe?

PATIENT: No. I didn't think she could do anything. I'm getting old and that's the price you pay. Do you think I should tell her?

NURSE: Yes, I do. Even if you two can't figure out why your hearing isn't as good as it was, she might be able to do something to help you hear better. I think she'd want to know.

PATIENT: Maybe I should. I'll let her know when I see her this afternoon.

The patient had already assessed this situation. In his opinion his situation would not be responsive to intervention and therefore there was no need to discuss it with the doctor. He acted on that assumption and did not present his problem for consultation until encouraged to do so.

These potential sources of conflict are aggravated by the concern that the patient and the health care provider do not use a common vocabulary. Indeed, in 1961 Samora, Saunders, and Larson presented research findings that suggested that "in any instance of practitioner-provider communication there is the possibility of misunderstanding or nonunderstanding on the part of the patient due to a vocabulary deficiency" (p. 92). In a similar vein, Mazzullo, Lasagna, and Griner (1974) found that "misinterpretation by patients of instructions on prescriptions may be an important factor in noncompliance with medication regimens" (p. 931). As a result, they urged clearer communication between patients and their providers about medication prescriptions.

The manner in which the patient perceives the health care provider may influence compliance. Falvo et al. (1980), in a study about physician-patient relationships, demonstrated that failure to comply was associated with the patient's perceptions that the doctor was not friendly or understanding about the patient's concern about the illness.

On the positive side, Becker and Maiman (1980) have demonstrated that adherence is greater when the patient's expectations have been fulfilled, when the provider asks about and respects all the patient's concerns, and when the patient and health care provider substantially agree on specifics of the regimen. Likewise, Falvo et al. (1980) noted that there was greater compliance if the patients perceived the physician as listening to their concerns, explaining their condition understandably, and considering their feelings and concerns when treatment was planned. Of note in other studies is the finding that problems acknowledged by both the patient and the practitioner were more likely to be reported as improved by the patient (DiMatteo, Prince, & Taranta, 1979; Starfield et al., 1981).

The system in which care is delivered can have a profound influence on the patient's perceptions of the health care provider. For example, Finnerty (1981) in his informal study found that the patients who withdrew from their hypertension follow-up had many complaints about the health care system. He noted that "their major complaints were long waiting times and the lack of patient-physician relationships at the clinic" (p. 82). In support of the patients' complaints Finnerty observed that the average amount of time actually spent with the physician was 7.5 minutes and that took place after a very long waiting period. In addition the patients often met with a different physician each visit. The system clearly did not support patient compliance.

Continuity of health care is likely to influence compliance with therapeutic regimens positively, as suggested. If patients see the same practitioners throughout a series of encounters, the resulting relationship may be stronger and more productive. In turn, patients may be more likely to follow prescribed regimens. This was confirmed by Becker, Drachman, and Kirscht (1974), who discovered that the extent to which mothers reported usually seeing the same physician correlated significantly ($p < .05$) with all the compliance variables (knowledge about the date of the follow-up appointment as well as about the medication and the number of times it was to be administered, administering the medication, and keeping the follow-up appointment). Satisfaction with the clinic was also predictive ($p < .05$) of administering the medication and keeping the follow-up appointment.

The relationship between the patient and the practitioner has an uncertain effect on eventual patient compliance. However, it is a variable over which the practitioner can exert some influence and therefore needs careful consideration when attempting to increase patient compliance. For example, one of the respondents to the authors' survey, when confronted with patient noncompliance, reported that her first response is "to further develop the patient-nurse relationship so that teaching can be given all the time—whether formally or informally."

Again, the relationship between the patient and the health care provider is one of the many variables in the patient compliance process. Other variables must also be considered.

EFFECT OF FAMILY AND FRIENDS

What effect do family and friends have on a patient's willingness to seek health care or undertake health-related activities? Although it is difficult to separate this factor from a variety of others, it is likely that social support plays an important part in patient compliance. This was acknowledged by the respondents to the authors' survey, 84 percent of whom indicated that noncompliance could be associated with lack of support from the patient's family or friends. Davis (1968) concurred, noting that family discord is closely associated with noncompliance.

The influence of family and friends can begin as early as the decision to seek medical advice. Most patients discuss their symptoms with someone else before seeking medical care. Patients usually follow the advice and recommendations that they received during this period. Mootz (1982) notes that "people who belong to cohesive networks with nonprofessional beliefs about medical care make the least use of medical services and vice versa" (p. 44).

Once medical care is obtained, the influence of family and friends continues. In a study of hemodialysis patients, Procci (1978) found that patients living with a spouse, children, or fiancée had a greater degree of dietary compliance than individuals with other living arrangements. In fact, 86 percent of the patients who had other living arrangements did not comply with their dietary restrictions. On the other hand, Becker, Drachman, and Kirscht (1974) were unable to demonstrate a relationship between illness or other problems in the mother's family and compliance with medications prescribed for the child's otitis media.

The influence of family and friends can either conflict with or support the health care provider's recommendations. It is important, when planning patient education, to assess the probable influence of the patient's family and friends on prescribed health behaviors. In this way, strategies can be developed to support the family and friends as well as the patient in fulfilling a treatment program.

The patients' families or other supports can and should be included in any planned strategies for education or for improved patient compliance with a therapeutic regimen. In many cases, such as with young children or patients who return to the community unable to care for themselves, it is the family who provides the care. In a very real sense, the family becomes the focus of compliance-improving strategies in these cases.

Even if the family members are not actually providing care to the patient, they have an influence on the patient's willingness and ability to fulfill a treatment regimen. Sackett et al. (1978) supported this relationship. They noted that a group of researchers at Johns Hopkins Hospital found that educating patients' families and urging them to support the treatment program resulted in a significant reduction in blood pressure for some patients.

When patients begin on a therapeutic regimen, there is often a simultaneous effect on their circle of family and friends. The degree to which the relationship between the patient, family, and friends is disrupted by the prescribed treatments also influences the patient's willingness to comply.

The bottom line is that the *patient* must actually comply. However, there is a strong case to continue and expand on assessing the influence and support of family members and friends in initial and ongoing patient assessments.

THE HEALTH BELIEF MODEL

One approach that has been used to explain and predict the health behavior of individuals is the Health Belief Model. The Health Belief Model is a framework that attempts to explain and correlate a variety of factors that influence a person's willingness to obtain health care and to comply with the resulting recommendations. It was originally developed to explain preventive health actions, but later work suggests that the Model may be useful in explaining behaviors in the presence of illness as well.

The Health Belief Model was developed in the early 1950s by Rosenstock and his colleagues. The Model also has its roots in the work of Kurt Lewin, who did much of the early work about field theory. The Health Belief Model is an example of the value-expectancy models that hypothesize that decisions about whether to take an action depend on:

- the value that individuals have placed on the outcome, and
- their estimate of the probability that a given action actually produces the outcome (Becker & Maiman, 1975).

The Health Belief Model consists of five key components that influence an individual's health behaviors. Those components, in the preventive health behavior context, are displayed in Figure 3–2. In this context, the Model proposes that individuals must believe that they are susceptible to the disease and that if they contracted it, the disease would have serious consequences on some aspects of life. These two elements are thought to establish individual readiness to take action, but the direction of that action is not predicted. An evaluation of the benefits of and barriers to the action then follows. Specifically individuals must believe that the intended actions would alleviate the problem and that barriers to the action can be overcome with reasonable effort. The fifth factor involves a cue to action, which appears "to serve to make the individual consciously aware of his feelings, thus enabling him to bring them to bear on the particular problem" (Becker & Maiman, 1975, p. 22). It is the manner in which the individual perceives these issues that is the basis for the Health Belief Model.

A case example illustrates some of the elements of the Health Belief Model. The patient, Mr. Sanders, is 40 years old and has been smoking for 17 years. He commented,

> The doctor tells me that I am prone to lung cancer because I smoke and because my father died of lung cancer. The doctor also said that the statistics show a higher rate of lung cancer in men and I believe him. I want to quit smoking because I don't want to die of lung cancer and I think not smoking will help. It won't be easy but I saw how sick my dad got. I'll really try this time and hopefully I can quit. Sign me up for the next Stop Smoking Program.

This man believed that he was susceptible to a condition, that the condition was serious, and that the prescribed action would help. All those factors are incorporated in the Health Belief Model.

In addition to the five elements, the individual's health motivations have been included in more recent versions of the Health Belief Model. Health motivations refer to the degree of interest in and concern about health matters in general (Becker & Maiman, 1980).

Various modifying factors are also part of the model. Those modifying factors include demographic information, structural factors (e.g., various aspects of the regimen), and attitudinal factors (about the provider and other aspects of the health care system). Interaction and enabling factors have been added as well. These factors would include prior experience with illness or the recommended action, the source of advice or referral, and the provider-patient relationship (Becker, 1974). It is assumed that these factors affect an individual's health motivations and perceptions, but that they are not direct causes of health behavior (Figure 3–2).

Figure 3–2 The Health Belief Model in the Preventive Context

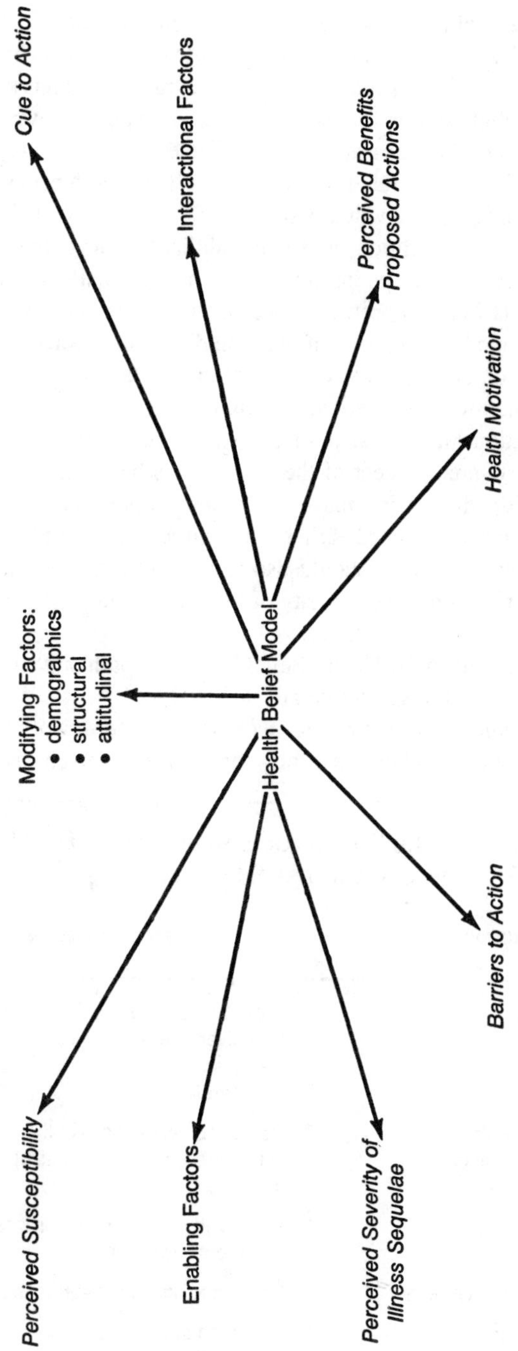

Although the Health Belief Model was originally developed to explain preventive health behavior, subsequent activities have sought to explain the behavior of those with known diseases or health conditions. Minimal modification is required to adapt the Health Belief Model for use in situations where known health problems exist. Those modifications are listed in Table 3–2. Basically, when illness situations exist, the Health Belief Model suggests that health behavior can be explained by examining the individual's beliefs in the accuracy of the diagnosis, resusceptibility to the condition, and vulnerability to other illnesses and illness in general (Becker, 1974). The importance of an individual's belief in the accuracy of the diagnosis was demonstrated by Becker, Drachman, and Kirscht (1972), who found that mothers' agreement with the diagnosis predicted knowledge about the medication and the follow-up appointment date as well as compliance with the medication regimen and actually keeping the follow-up appointment. This relationship was also supported by the respondents to the authors' survey. Seventy-three percent of the respondents believed that the patients' lack of belief in the diagnosis contributes to noncompliance.

Some of the other elements included earlier in the discussion about the Health Belief Model (in a preventive context) should also be altered somewhat to apply to illness states. For example, perceived severity of the illness relates to the illness that the patient has contracted (Figure 3–2).

The five major components of the Health Belief Model, in both preventive and illness contexts, are explained in greater detail.

1. *Perceived susceptibility to a disease or belief in the accuracy of the diagnosis.* Do individuals actually believe that they can contract a given disease or

Table 3–2 A Comparison of the Five Major Elements of the Health Belief Model in Preventive and Illness Situations

Preventive Situations	*Presence of Illness*
1. Perceived susceptibility	1. Belief in the accuracy of the diagnosis Perceived resusceptibility Perceived susceptibility to disease in general
2. Perceived seriousness of the consequences of the illness or condition	2. Perceived seriousness of the consequences of the illness or condition
3. Perceived benefits of proposed preventive action	3. Perceived benefits of the proposed therapeutic regimen
4. Barriers to action are surmountable	4. Barriers to action are surmountable
5. Presence of a cue to action	5. Presence of a cue to action

condition? Do they believe that the diagnosis is accurate? Do they believe that they are susceptible to contracting the problem again in the future? This element, if it is present, can range from low to high perceived susceptibility.

The idea of perceived susceptibility has gained support in various research studies. For example, Becker, Drachman, and Kirscht (1974) discovered that mothers who felt that their children were susceptible to another bout of otitis media were more likely to administer the prescribed antibiotics and to keep follow-up appointments.

2. *Belief that the disease would have or will have serious consequences on some aspect of life.* This component implies that the individual considers the question "What would happen if I were to really come down with this disease or problem?" Evaluation incorporates factors other than health. Individuals consider whether the disease will affect their ability to work or to carry out other aspects of their usual daily lives. Economic issues are considered as well. The effects of the condition on their families or others close to them are also considered.

Again, a range of perceived serious consequences can be considered. Individuals may consider the consequences to be mild or severe.

Research support has been determined for this element of the Health Belief Model. In the Becker, Drachman, and Kirscht (1974) study cited, mothers who believed that otitis media is a serious illness were significantly more likely to comply with the therapeutic regimen ($p <.05$).

3. *Belief that the proposed action will reduce susceptibility to the condition or be effective in controlling the current problem.* In other words, the person expects that the behavior will lead to desired health outcomes. On the other hand, the proposed actions may be perceived as ineffective. A classic example was found in a *Boston Globe* article focusing on health. This article reported the results of a study relating cholesterol levels and heart attacks. One of the researchers, Goor, commented: "To get people to modify a habit, especially a 'habit' as pleasurable as eating, requires a high degree of motivation. First they have to believe that it will actually do some good" (Knox, 1984, p. 41). The practitioners responding to the authors' survey agreed that this is an important factor in patient compliance. Seventy-six percent believed that noncompliance could be related to the patient's beliefs that the regimen is not helpful.

4. *Barriers to the proposed action perceived as surmountable.* This component is related to the perceived cost of the action and the person's estimate of the amount of effort necessary to overcome any perceived barriers to undertaking the action. The barriers may be real or perceived. They may also be generated by internal or external sources. For example, the person may decide internally that there is too much effort involved in following health directions to stop smoking or lose weight. External barriers to action would include such factors as a drug store that is an inconvenient distance away for prescriptions or physical therapy appointments that conflict with a job that provides a much needed salary.

5. *Existence of a concomitant cue to action.* As noted, this cue helps make the individual aware of feelings, allowing them to influence the particular problem. The cue may arise from internal or external sources. Internal cues may result from a changing body function such as pain or disability. External cues may result from the knowledge that someone else has contracted a disease. For example, the knowledge that a close friend or colleague succumbed to a myocardial infarction may provide a cue for contemporaries to undergo a medical examination. Another example evolved when a number of women sought breast examinations after Betty Ford's and Happy Rockefeller's radical mastectomies became public knowledge.

The intensity of the required cue to action appears to depend on differences in the level of readiness to take action (Rosenstock, 1974). Those who do not perceive that they are susceptible to disease require a strong stimulus or cue to action. Individuals who already believe that they are likely to contract the disease may be stimulated by a very weak cue to action.

Various assumptions are involved in the Health Belief Model. The Health Belief Model assumes that the person perceives illness as undesirable and to be avoided and, further, that an illness-free state is preferred. It also assumes that persons are rational, especially in the context of obtaining health care (Fabrega, 1973). It assumes that individuals evaluate instances of illness using economic or utility considerations and make a decision about which optimal action will eliminate the problem (Baric, 1969).

What sort of support has been demonstrated for the Health Belief Model through research activities? The findings have been diverse and at times conflictive. This can be observed in the selected results reported next.

Kirscht and Rosenstock (1977) found that patients with higher levels of personal susceptibility were more likely to adhere to the treatment regimen for their hypertension. Perceived severity of stroke and heart or kidney disease was also associated with compliance although not at the significant level. Furthermore, they found that higher scores on belief in the effectiveness of medical interventions were related to medication but not dietary compliance.

Vertinsky et al. (1976) studied compliance with a Tay-Sachs screening program. They found that perceived seriousness of the condition was predictive of attendance at the screening program. Attendees also tended to believe that they could be carrying the trait and that determining whether or not they were would be beneficial as they made decisions about family planning.

Becker, Drachman, and Kirscht (1972) reported that mothers who felt that their children contract illnesses easily and often and who saw illness as an important threat to children in general were also more likely to keep appointments and to administer medications. Mothers who believed that their children were susceptible to ear infections were also more likely to comply with appointments and medication schedules. The mothers' perceptions regarding the severity of the illness predicted compliance with medication but not with appointment keeping.

Andreöli (1981) concluded that for male hypertensive patients self-concept and health beliefs are not different in those who comply with prescribed therapy from beliefs in those who do not comply.

Stillman (1977) found that although 97 percent of her subjects scored high in perceived benefits and 87 percent scored high in perceived susceptibility, only 40 percent of the women studied did monthly self-breast examinations. She noted that it is difficult to conclude that beliefs cause behavior in this situation.

Ferguson and Bole (1979) studied 40 patients with rheumatoid arthritis. Their only statistically significant finding for noncompliance with aspirin and exercise was a lack of patient belief in benefits of the actions.

Cummings et al. (1982) studied 116 patients and their compliance with the various elements of a hemodialysis regimen. Those elements included fluid restrictions, dietary restrictions, and phosphorus-binding medications. They evaluated the patient compliance using two measures. First, they used patient self-reports. Then, they used objective data available in the patients' charts (e.g., weights and blood chemistry determinations). The researchers found that beliefs about benefits were significantly correlated with both self-reported and chart data about phosphorus-binding medication; strongly correlated with self-report about diet; and moderately correlated with chart data about diet. The number of barriers reported significantly and negatively correlated with compliance for each element.

In summary, research conducted about the Health Belief Model has produced diverse findings. Many of the findings showed a relationship between one or more elements of the model. Others could not produce a significant, positive relationship. However, the findings are such that continuing research about the model is appropriate.

How useful is the Health Belief Model in the patient education process? It can be very beneficial. First, it emphasizes the importance of the individual's perceptions in the health behavior process. It also outlines some very influential factors that can help explain the health behavior of individuals. Finally, the Health Belief Model points to the interrelatedness of various factors that influence health behaviors. Other factors also influence patient compliance; one is studied in the next section.

LOCUS OF CONTROL

NURSE: Mr. White, that sore on your foot looks infected. Is it sore?

PATIENT: No, it's not too bad. It looks worse than it feels.

NURSE: Did you have trouble doing the special care for your feet that we talked about the last time you visited me?

PATIENT: No, I haven't had trouble but I didn't figure it would do anything. If you're going to have trouble, you'll have trouble. It's God's will.

This conversation is not an unusual one. The patient believes that a prescribed activity will not prevent a problem because if an individual is fated to have the problem, it will occur. In this belief system, nothing that the patient can do will prevent the problem from occurring. More specifically, this patient believes that a deity or outside force controls some very significant aspects of life. Most practitioners come in contact with individuals holding this belief many times in their practice. Practitioners may observe that the individuals who believe that they have little control over their lives contrast sharply with another group who believe that they can control their lives. A conversation with an individual in the latter group will proceed along very different lines.

NURSE: Mrs. Hampshire, it's good to see you and you look wonderful! How are you feeling?

PATIENT: I'm feeling a lot better than when I was in the hospital with my heart attack. It really helps to get home because I'm so much more comfortable there.

NURSE: You look as though you've lost weight, too.

PATIENT: Well, I decided that if I am going to get better and stay that way, I have to get busy and lose weight. I'm also getting the exercise the nurses and doctors told me about while I was in the hospital. You know, the Lord helps those who help themselves.

A significant difference in these two situations is the individual's perceptions of how much control the person has over life's events. Of equal significance is the fact that the individuals subsequently undertook very different behaviors. Mrs. Hampshire, believing that her activities would positively influence outcomes, followed dietary and exercise prescriptions. On the other hand, Mr. White, believing that his condition was in God's hands, did not carry out diabetic foot care as prescribed. The observations made in these two conversations are consistent as groups of individuals are studied. The study of these beliefs is conducted under the topic of locus of control.

Locus of control is a psychosocial construct that proposes that a relationship exists between an individual's perceptions of control over outcomes and the likelihood of taking specific actions. It is derived from Rotter's social learning theory, which holds, in part, that individuals have a choice in how they will behave. Like the Health Belief Model, locus of control is another example of the value-expectancy models.

Locus of control asks if individuals perceive a contingency relationship between their behaviors and associated reinforcers, rewards, or events. (In the patient education context, the focus is on patients and their willingness to undertake health actions.) More specifically, locus of control suggests that when a person perceives rewards, punishments, or results as contingent on personal actions, behavior is quite different than when such reinforcements are believed to occur independently of efforts. Locus of control further hypothesizes that learning differs when individuals perceive that they control the contingency between their behaviors and reinforcements compared to when they do not perceive this relationship.

In examining the relationship between behaviors and outcomes, a continuum is established. At one end are those individuals who perceive a causal relationship between their behavior and the outcomes. These individuals are said to be at the *internal* end of the scale. The *external* end of the scale is reserved for individuals who do not see such a contingency relationship but instead attribute outcomes to an external force. They may cite luck, chance, or a deity as the underlying force (Rotter, 1966).

The characteristics or traits of externals and internals appear to differ in a variety of ways. For example, because externals do not see a relationship between their own actions and the resulting effects, these statements seem to be supported:

- Externals possess little information that is useful in achieving relevant health goals. In addition, they do not attempt to obtain information (Phares, 1976).
- Externals generalize less from the past and cannot use increasing experience on a current task to develop better methods of handling the situation or to establish more accurate expectancies (Phares, 1976).
- They are susceptible to influence, especially when they feel it is coming from someone of status. They conform to the judgments of others more readily (Phares, 1976).
- Externals exhibit little capacity to delay gratification (Lefcourt, 1982).
- Externals may not try because they do not believe that their efforts are effective (MacDonald, 1972).

On the other hand, internals believe themselves to be in control of their own destinies. As a result, these statements seem to be supported:

- Internals actively acquire more knowledge about their problems or the task before them. Therefore, they are in a better position to deal with the problems or tasks at hand (Dabbs & Kirscht, 1978).
- "Internals will resist the efforts of others to manipulate them" but will use and benefit from assistance from authority figures (Phares, 1976, p. 80).
- They can cope better with potentially threatening situations (MacDonald, 1972).
- Internals can focus on long-term gains and forego more immediate rewards to achieve them (Lefcourt, 1982).
- They can understand and perceive a relationship between behavior and results. For example, they are more likely to perceive their attempts at preventive behavior as diminishing their vulnerability to illness.

An individual's locus of control orientation is an enduring and stable characteristic. Many factors, however, can contribute to the direction of one's locus of control orientation. For example, those in lower socioeconomic classes, minority groups, and with physical disabilities tend to be more external (MacDonald, 1972). Lefcourt (1982) also observed that age affects locus orientation in that the young tend to be more external. He noted that significant life events can effect a change in locus of control orientation. The crisis of illness is one life event that can produce a change in locus of control orientation, generally toward the more external end of the continuum. Schillinger (1983) noted that many situations involved with illness cannot be controlled. This reality can lead to extreme externality. There is inconsistency in these observations, however. For example, McCusker and Morrow (1979) were unable to establish a relationship between age, sex, marital status, and locus of control orientation. When health was examined within the locus of control context, Lau (1982) found that practicing a variety of different health habits as a child was associated with beliefs in the controllability of health. Of concern was his finding that experiences with sickness in one's family tend to lead one to believe that health is not controllable and that self-care efforts are not effective. Further study is needed to confirm the precedents of locus of control orientation.

It should be emphasized that rarely, if ever, are individuals purely internal or external. Rather, most will fall somewhere along the continuum between the two dimensions.

There has been a significant amount of research regarding locus of control. Some of the findings are very pertinent to health education and the study of health behaviors. As has been the case with other studies regarding health behavior, the findings are at times conflictive. Some of the findings are summarized next.

When studying the relationship of locus of control to learning, Seeman and Evans (1962) found support for a relationship between an external locus of control and poor learning. Externals were found to have significantly lower scores on tests for objective knowledge.

Those who are chronically disabled appear to have a tendency toward externality. An example of this was described in a study of suicide in chronic hemodialysis patients. The suicide rate among hemodialysis patients was 400 times that of the general population. The investigators postulated that because chronic dialysis patients tend to have an external locus of control, they do not perceive their actions to be life-sustaining (Goldstein & Reznikoff, 1971).

Bollin and Hart (1982) noted that "those subjects who perceived that a health related reward was contingent upon their own behavior were more compliant than those who felt the health related rewards were more controlled by forces outside themselves" (p. 45). McCusker and Morrow found that internal women were more likely to do self-breast examinations (1979).

Patients who were more internal were more likely to comply with medication regimens than were those who attributed outcomes to chance, according to research conducted by Kirscht and Rosenstock (1977) with 132 hypertensive patients. Likewise, MacDonald (1970) found that internals were more likely to attempt pregnancy control. The results, however, were not confirmed at a level of significance.

Because internals appear to be more capable of handling difficult situations (such as illnesses), techniques have been developed to help external individuals to become more internally focused. Techniques are being developed that might help those who tend to be externally focused become more internal. Those techniques include

- Helping the individual to see the situation in a new light through discussions and confrontation. In this way the person has alternative ways to analyze situations.
- Assisting the person to develop skills in problem solving. In this technique the emphasis is on new behaviors and not necessarily a change in attitude.
- Challenging external statements and rewarding internal ones.
- Helping the person focus on the outcomes of personal behavior, emphasizing the relationship between the two. This technique challenges individuals to assess what could have been done differently to change the results of past problems, how current problems can be approached in a different manner, and how future situations will be handled (MacDonald, 1972).

These questions and techniques are designed to help individuals see themselves as having some power to affect outcomes or events in their lives, a characteristic more usually associated with internal individuals.

Locus of control orientation can be measured in various ways. Rotter developed the initial measurement scale, and it has been used in many studies. Rotter's locus of control scale is included in Exhibit 3–1. Wallston, Wallston, Kaplan, and Maides (1976) developed a health locus of control scale. That scale is found in Exhibit 3–2.

Although the research findings are not conclusive, there is significant support for assessing a patient's locus of control orientation. In doing so, the practitioner may begin to develop supportive strategies for patients at various points along the internal-external continuum. Obviously, locus of control is not the only factor involved in health behaviors. Other factors influencing compliance must also be examined.

Exhibit 3–1 Rotter's Locus of Control Scale

Instructions. This is a questionnaire to find out the way in which certain important events in our society affect different people. Each item consists of a pair of alternatives lettered *a* or *b*. Please select the one statement of each pair (*and only one*) which you more strongly *believe* to be the case as far as you're concerned. Be sure to select the one you actually *believe* to be more true rather than the one you would like to be true. This is a measure of personal belief: obviously there are no right or wrong answers.

1. ____ a. Children get into trouble because their parents punish them too much.
   ____ b. The trouble with most children nowadays is that their parents are too easy with them.

2. ____ a. Many of the unhappy things in people's lives are partly due to bad luck.
   ____ b. People's misfortunes result from the mistakes they make.

3. ____ a. One of the major reasons why we have wars is because people don't take enough interest in politics.
   ____ b. There will always be wars, no matter how hard people try to prevent them.

4. ____ a. In the long run, people get the respect they deserve in this world.
   ____ b. Unfortunately, an individual's worth often passes unrecognized no matter how hard he tries.

5. ____ a. The idea that teachers are unfair to students is nonsense.
   ____ b. Most students don't realize the extent to which their grades are influenced by accidental happenings.

6. ____ a. Without the right breaks one cannot be an effective leader.
   ____ b. Capable people who fail to become leaders have not taken advantage of their opportunities.

7. ____ a. No matter how hard you try some people just don't like you.
   ____ b. People who can't get others to like them don't understand how to get along with others.

8. ____ a. Heredity plays the major role in determining one's personality.
   ____ b. It is one's experiences in life which determine what one is like.

9. ____ a. I have often found that what is going to happen will happen.
   ____ b. Trusting in fate has never turned out as well for me as making a decision to take a definite course of action.

10. ____ a. In the case of the well prepared student there is rarely if ever such a thing as an unfair test.
    ____ b. Many times exam questions tend to be so unrelated to course work that studying is really useless.

11. ____ a. Becoming a success is a matter of hard work, luck has little or nothing to do with it.
    ____ b. Getting a good job depends mainly on being in the right place at the right time.

12. ____ a. The average citizen can have an influence in government decisions.
    ____ b. The world is run by the few people in power and there is not much the little guy can do about it.

Exhibit 3–1 continued

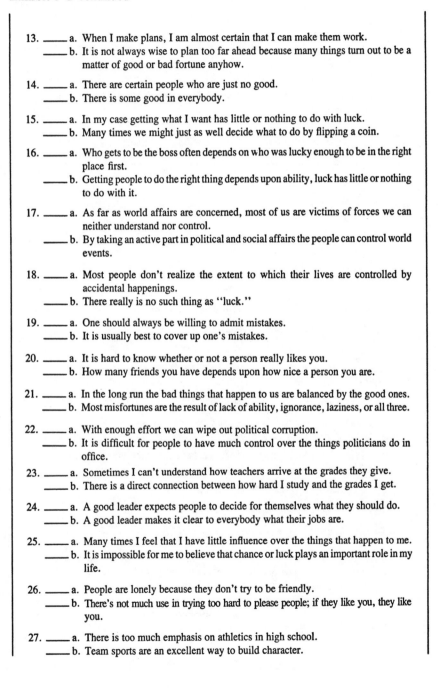

13. ____ a. When I make plans, I am almost certain that I can make them work.
 ____ b. It is not always wise to plan too far ahead because many things turn out to be a matter of good or bad fortune anyhow.

14. ____ a. There are certain people who are just no good.
 ____ b. There is some good in everybody.

15. ____ a. In my case getting what I want has little or nothing to do with luck.
 ____ b. Many times we might just as well decide what to do by flipping a coin.

16. ____ a. Who gets to be the boss often depends on who was lucky enough to be in the right place first.
 ____ b. Getting people to do the right thing depends upon ability, luck has little or nothing to do with it.

17. ____ a. As far as world affairs are concerned, most of us are victims of forces we can neither understand nor control.
 ____ b. By taking an active part in political and social affairs the people can control world events.

18. ____ a. Most people don't realize the extent to which their lives are controlled by accidental happenings.
 ____ b. There really is no such thing as "luck."

19. ____ a. One should always be willing to admit mistakes.
 ____ b. It is usually best to cover up one's mistakes.

20. ____ a. It is hard to know whether or not a person really likes you.
 ____ b. How many friends you have depends upon how nice a person you are.

21. ____ a. In the long run the bad things that happen to us are balanced by the good ones.
 ____ b. Most misfortunes are the result of lack of ability, ignorance, laziness, or all three.

22. ____ a. With enough effort we can wipe out political corruption.
 ____ b. It is difficult for people to have much control over the things politicians do in office.

23. ____ a. Sometimes I can't understand how teachers arrive at the grades they give.
 ____ b. There is a direct connection between how hard I study and the grades I get.

24. ____ a. A good leader expects people to decide for themselves what they should do.
 ____ b. A good leader makes it clear to everybody what their jobs are.

25. ____ a. Many times I feel that I have little influence over the things that happen to me.
 ____ b. It is impossible for me to believe that chance or luck plays an important role in my life.

26. ____ a. People are lonely because they don't try to be friendly.
 ____ b. There's not much use in trying too hard to please people; if they like you, they like you.

27. ____ a. There is too much emphasis on athletics in high school.
 ____ b. Team sports are an excellent way to build character.

Exhibit 3–1 continued

28. _____ a. What happens to me is my own doing.
_____ b. Sometimes I feel that I don't have enough control over the direction my life is taking.

29. _____ a. Most of the time I can't understand why politicians behave the way they do.
_____ b. In the long run the people are responsible for bad government on a national as well as on a local level.

Source: "Generalized Expectancies for Internal versus External Control of Reinforcement" [entire issue], by J.B. Rotter, 1966, *Psychological Monographs 80* (609). Copyright 1966 by the American Psychological Association.

Exhibit 3–2 Health Locus of Control Scale

Item	*Direction**
1. If I take care of myself, I can avoid illness.	I
2. Whenever I get sick it is because of something I've done or not done.	I
3. Good health is largely a matter of good fortune.	E
4. No matter what I do, if I am going to get sick I will get sick.	E
5. Most people do not realize the extent to which their illnesses are controlled by accidental happenings.	E
6. I can only do what my doctor tells me to do.	E
7. There are so many strange diseases around that you can never know how or when you might pick one up.	E
8. When I feel ill, I know it is because I have not been getting the proper exercise or eating right.	I
9. People who never get sick are just plain lucky.	E
10. People's ill health results from their own carelessness.	I
11. I am directly responsible for my health.	I

*I = internally worded, E = externally worded. The scale is scored in the external direction, with each item scored from 1 (strongly disagree) to 6 (strongly agree) for the externally worded items and reverse scored for the internally worded items.

Source: "Development and Validation of the Health Locus of Control (HLC) Scale," by B.S. Wallston, K.A. Wallston, G.D. Kaplan, and S.A. Maides, 1976, *Journal of Consulting and Clinical Psychology, 44*(4), 581. Copyright 1976 by the American Psychological Association.

THE PATIENT'S VALUES

The values that individuals hold about health and related issues greatly affect their willingness to seek care and to follow therapeutic recommendations. Health care providers are very aware of this factor. Eighty-three percent of the practitioners responding to the authors' survey indicated that they believed noncompliance could be attributed to patient values about health differing from those held by the practitioners. Because of the critical relationship between values and health behaviors, it is important that those involved in health education be aware of the possible effects of values. This section defines values and explores how they may influence the process of patient education.

The rationale for studying values is extensive. Suchman (1970) suggests that "values, attitudes and personality exert an important influence on how man perceives, interprets and responds to illness" (p. 105). Goldstein (1959) adds further credibility to the study of values when he comments that "the behavior of patients (can) be understood only if it is considered as determined by a definite value and . . . we can help the patient only when we take account of this value" (p. 179). It is quite clear that values are an important adjunct to understanding the health behaviors of individuals.

Such an understanding can begin with an explanation of values and a description of their nature. Rokeach (1973) has done much of the work in this area, and he categorizes values as a type of belief. Values serve as criteria or standards for the purpose of making evaluations. Unlike attitudes, values are not linked to specific objects or situations; rather, they are abstract ideals. In fact, values transcend specific objects and situations. A value, then, is an enduring single belief that one behavior or goal is preferable (personally or socially) to another. In other words, values represent a person's beliefs about ideal modes of conduct and ideal terminal goals. Based on these descriptions, two types of values can be identified: (1) instrumental (concerned with ideal modes of conduct) and (2) terminal (concerned with end states of existence).

The number of values held by an individual is quite small when compared to the almost endless number of possible beliefs. Values can be placed on a continuum or arranged in a hierarchical organization. The organization of values is in the form of a value system. Each instrumental and terminal value can evolve into a system with a hierarchical ordering of the values within it. In fact, it is conceivable that an individual could be in a situation in which various values are incongruent. Rokeach (1980) suggests that, in those cases, the individual's value system is a "learned organization of rules for making choices and for resolving conflicts between two or more modes of behavior or between two or more end states of existence" (p. 161).

Values may have several other functions. Rokeach (1980) points out that

> once a value is internalized it becomes, consciously or unconsciously, a standard or criterion for guiding action, for developing and maintaining attitudes toward relevant objects and situations, for justifying one's own and others' actions and attitudes, for morally judging self and others, and for comparing self with others. Finally a value is a standard employed to influence the values, attitudes and actions of at least some others—one's children's, for example. (p. 160)

It is helpful to acknowledge that values may not be applied consistently. For example, people may apply values in one way to themselves but another way to others. In a sense, the adage "Do as I say, not as I do" reflects an example of how values might be applied in different ways.

How does this information influence the process of patient education? Values about health are one component of the patient's total system of values. Although it is sometimes difficult to acknowledge or understand, in many situations health values are not a priority in an individual's value hierarchy. In fact, other values or attitudes may conflict at times with those about health. As Gillum and Barsky (1974) acknowledge:

> Each patient faces a wide array of competing demands for his time, money, energy and attention. Health care is only one of these and some estimation of the others is helpful in detecting those who will not comply subsequently. Compliance, from the patient's viewpoint, is really a series of tradeoffs in which the patient gives up or takes on certain behaviors in return for promised benefits. (p. 1566)

A significant body of information has been gathered about the way in which values influence behaviors. Much of that information is incorporated in value-expectancy models. Those models generally assert that behavior is the result of the *value* that an individual places on the outcome of an action and the individual's *expectation* that the action will indeed lead to the desired outcome. The Health Belief Model and the locus of control construct are two examples of value-expectancy model application to health situations.

Wallston, Maides, and Wallston (1976) incorporated health values in their research about health-related information seeking. Their study involved 88 college students who were told that they were assisting a new hypertension clinic select appropriate pamphlets for its patients. The subjects were given a list of titles and authors of hypertension pamphlets and asked to indicate the ones that they would choose if visiting the clinic. The subjects also completed a health-related locus of control scale, a value survey, and a quiz on hypertension. The researchers hypothesized that "given the opportunity to gather information about a health problem which may or may not affect him/her, the internal who values health highly will seek more information than the one who does not value health or who holds external beliefs'' (p. 221). That hypothesis was supported at a significant ($p <.05$) level, leading the researchers to conclude that information seeking is a function of expectancy and value.

Other than the study just discussed, there is scant research about the specific effect of values on health behaviors. This is an area where significant contributions could be made. Rokeach developed a values survey for use in research (Exhibit 3–3). It does not specifically include health as a value; however, it can easily be modified to do so. The researchers involved in the study about information seeking extracted values from the Rokeach survey and added a value regarding health.

Values ultimately influence behaviors, including health-related behaviors. Health educators need to investigate the structure of their patients' value systems. It may be as simple as asking patients what is important to them in their lives. Continued research efforts may contribute to the development of an efficient, accurate mechanism for assessing this factor. In the interim, practitioners should assess their own values vis-à-vis those of their patients. In this way the potential for conflicting values can be evaluated and acknowledged. One of the responses to the authors' survey demonstrated a high level of understanding of differing values. The respondent indicated that, unlike the situation early in her career, ''I now feel comfortable with the fact that not everyone perceives health and healthy behaviors as a priority or even as a necessity.'' This is important because of the effect that conflicting values can have on patient compliance, as discussed in the section on the patient-provider relationship. Values, then, can influence compliance. Other factors may also be involved.

ATTRIBUTION AND HEALTH BEHAVIOR

The following conversation took place in a clinic waiting room between an obese, short-of-breath patient and her friend. The patient had just returned to the waiting room from the nurse's office.

PATIENT: My blood pressure is up again. The nurse said that it's higher than it usually is.

FRIEND: I'll bet it was the cab ride over that did it. You know how upset you were about the wild ride. And then you had to walk so far to get here. You're not used to walking that far.

PATIENT: No. I wasn't that upset about the cab ride, not enough to make my blood pressure go up so much. I think it was because I've gotten so much bad news this week. It seems like I've spent the week on the telephone hearing about people who are sick or dying. I'll bet that's what did it.

Exhibit 3–3 The Rokeach Value Survey

Instructions: Study the list carefully and pick out the one value which is the most important to you. Peel it off and paste it in Box 1 on the left. Then pick out the value which is second most important to you. Peel it off and paste it in Box 2. Then do the same for each of the remaining values. The value which is least important to you goes in Box 18. Work slowly and think carefully. If you change your mind, feel free to change your answers. The labels peel off easily and can be moved from place to place. The end result should truly show how you really feel. On the next page are 18 values listed in alphabetical order. Arrange them in order of importance to YOU, as guiding principles in YOUR life.

1 ______________________	A COMFORTABLE LIFE (a prosperous life)
2 ______________________	AN EXCITING LIFE (a stimulating, active life)
3 ______________________	A SENSE OF ACCOMPLISHMENT (lasting contribution)
4 ______________________	A WORLD AT PEACE (free of war and conflict)
5 ______________________	A WORLD OF BEAUTY (beauty of nature and the arts)
6 ______________________	EQUALITY (brotherhood, equal opportunity for all)
7 ______________________	FAMILY SECURITY (taking care of loved ones)
8 ______________________	FREEDOM (independence, free choice)
9 ______________________	HAPPINESS (contentedness)
10 ______________________	INNER HARMONY (freedom from inner conflict)
11 ______________________	MATURE LOVE (sexual and spiritual intimacy)
12 ______________________	NATIONAL SECURITY (protection from attack)
13 ______________________	PLEASURE (an enjoyable, leisurely life)
14 ______________________	SALVATION (saved, eternal life)
15 ______________________	SELF-RESPECT (self-esteem)
16 ______________________	SOCIAL RECOGNITION (respect, admiration)
17 ______________________	TRUE FRIENDSHIP (close companionship)
18 ______________________	WISDOM (a mature understanding of life)

Exhibit 3–3 continued

Below is another list of 18 values. Arrange them in order of importance, the same as before.

1 ______________	AMBITIOUS (hard-working, aspiring)
2 ______________	BROADMINDED (open-minded)
3 ______________	CAPABLE (competent, effective)
4 ______________	CHEERFUL (lighthearted, joyful)
5 ______________	CLEAN (neat, tidy)
6 ______________	COURAGEOUS (standing up for your beliefs)
7 ______________	FORGIVING (willing to pardon others)
8 ______________	HELPFUL (working for the welfare of others)
9 ______________	HONEST (sincere, truthful)
10 ______________	IMAGINATIVE (daring, creative)
11 ______________	INDEPENDENT (self-reliant, self-sufficient)
12 ______________	INTELLECTUAL (intelligent, reflective)
13 ______________	LOGICAL (consistent, rational)
14 ______________	LOVING (affectionate, tender)
15 ______________	OBEDIENT (dutiful, respectful)
16 ______________	POLITE (courteous, well-mannered)
17 ______________	RESPONSIBLE (dependable, reliable)
18 ______________	SELF-CONTROLLED (restrained, self-disciplined)

Source: Reprinted with permission of The Free Press, a Division of Macmillan, Inc., and *Halgren Tests from the Nature of Human Values* by M. Rokeach. Copyright © 1973 by The Free Press and Halgren Tests.

Most health practitioners would acknowledge that when patients are told that they have a disease or condition, they seek an answer to the question "why?" or "what caused it?" The need to know why or to understand the causes of life's events appears to be an inherent human trait. Through careful listening, one can detect this phenomenon in everyday life. For example, comments about how a back injury occurred ("I lifted the baby in a hurry") or about the origins of a cold ("I got wet last Thursday night when it was so chilly") are commonplace. In fact, the recent popularity of macrobiotic diets is at least partially based on a belief that cancer has diet-related causes.

The cause ascribed to an event (health-related or otherwise) is known as *attribution*, more specifically an *attribution of causality*. Attribution theory emerged from the study of individuals as they attempt to determine the causes of events in their lives. It has its foundations in the idea that individuals seek causes for events in their lives and in the lives of others. The study of attributions, including those in health-related situations, has as its goal to understand the perceptions that lay individuals have about the causes of their health problems. Attribution theory assumes that the act of ascribing causality to events has usefulness to individuals because it helps fulfill the need to explain, to predict, and, ultimately, to have some control over the events in their lives (Shaver, 1975).

The usefulness in studying attributions lies in the hypothesis that "future behaviors are, in part, determined by perceived causes of past events" (Weiner, 1974, p. 55). This implies that individuals will select a health behavior based on their perceptions of the cause of the problem. For example, a man experiencing chest pain will react differently if he perceives the cause of the pain to be chronic indigestion than if he believes that his symptoms are those of a myocardial infarction. Likewise, a woman who develops a persistent headache may pursue one course of action if she believes her headache to be the result of tension. Her behaviors may be very different if she perceives her headache to be the result of a tumor.

An attributional case example involves Julia, a newborn with multiple congenital anomalies. Julia's parents expressed the belief that her anomalies were caused by something they did (or failed to do) during the pregnancy. Consequently they felt that nothing they did would improve the situation. Therefore they did not complete most of the aspects of the treatment plan.

The basic process involved in ascribing a cause to an event is relatively simple (Figure 3–3). The individual perceives a stimulus or event, in the health context a symptom or alteration in bodily functioning. A label or definition is given to the event, and the individual then attempts to establish its cause. The cause established is proposed to have a direct or indirect influence on future beliefs or behaviors.

Although the process appears simple, many intervening factors can influence the attribution process. Some of those factors are included in Figure 3–4. The individual's previous experiences affect the causes ascribed to a current event. Likewise, the individual's assumptions, expectations, attitudes, and values influence the type of attributions made. As individuals attempt to determine the cause of their health problem, they often gather information from a variety of sources, including friends, family, the media, or health care providers. The information

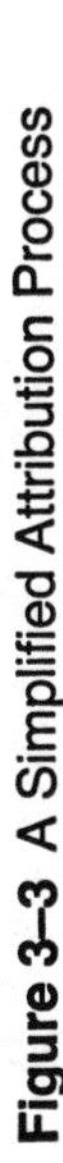

Figure 3–3 A Simplified Attribution Process

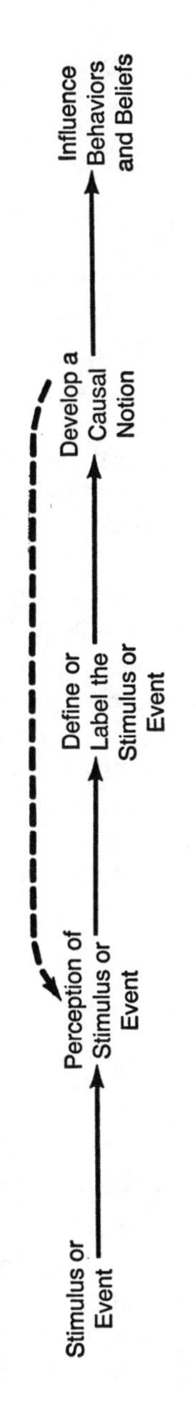

Figure 3–4 Factors Influencing the Attribution Process

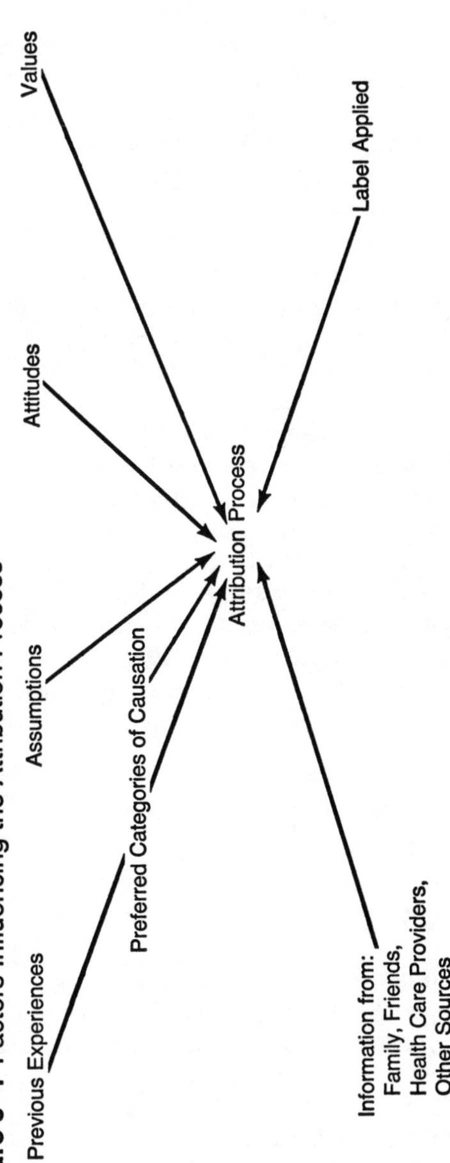

gathered provides direction to the attribution ascribed and, ultimately, to the individual's response. Some researchers have observed that individuals develop patterns or categories of attributions, another intervening factor influencing the attribution process.

In the process of formulating causal explanations, the application of a label to the event is of major significance. There seems to be agreement that the label given, or the way in which an event is described, has a profound impact on the cause assigned. This also suggests that the actions taken will depend, at least in part, on the label attached to the phenomenon. The appearance of unusual body sensations or symptoms seems to trigger a search for labels (Leventhal & Hirschman, 1982). Lau and Hartman's (1983) research provides support for the importance of labeling in that 37 percent and 49 percent of their subjects labeled their diseases, although they were not specifically asked to do so.

The search for labels is necessarily constrained by the individual's available repertoire. That repertoire may be sophisticated or basic, general or specific. The explanation that evolves will parallel the sophistication or generality of the label applied (Kanouse, 1972).

The close relationship between labels and attributions is further demonstrated by Kanouse's observation that the language used in the label usually contains implicit attributions (1972). Blaxter (1983) supported this observation in her study, which revealed that of 587 named diseases, 432 were labeled in a way suggesting their causes. As a result, the process of selecting a label for a bodily sensation often focuses the individual toward certain causes and away from others. This is not meant to imply that labeling always precedes assigning an attribution. Indeed, Morris and Kanouse (1979) suggest that the selection of a label can be influenced by the individual's causal assumptions about the symptom or feeling.

Several dimensions are associated with attributions. Some of them are

- locus of causality,
- stability,
- controllability,
- intentionality, and
- globality.

The locus of causality refers to the individual's perceptions about the origin of the problem. A locus range has internal attributions at one end and external at the other, and perceptions of causality can fall at any point on the continuum. Those who assign an internal cause to an event perceive themselves as contributing to the event. An external cause signifies that individuals perceive the event to be caused by an agent or factor external to them. Bulman and Wortman (1977) included locus of causality in their investigation of 29 spinal cord–injured patients. Their findings suggest that those patients who blame themselves for the injury-producing accident are more likely to cope in a positive manner than patients who attribute the cause of the accident to others.

Stability, or relative endurance, refers to the individual's beliefs about whether the cause is likely to change over time. Again, a range of possibilities from stable to unstable forms a continuum, and the attribution can be placed at any point along that continuum. Kelley (1967) proposes situations in which assigned causality is likely to be unstable. He notes that instability is likely to be high for the person who has

- little social support,
- prior information that is poor or ambiguous, and
- problems that are difficult and beyond one's capabilities.

These are conditions that patients frequently experience, and it is helpful for health educators to be aware of them.

Control is another causal dimension, and it deals with whether individuals believe that they have control over the assigned causes. As in locus of causality, the spectrum of locus of control has internality at one end and externality at the other, with assigned causality placed anywhere along the continuum. Locus of control examines whether the individual perceives self or external agents to be the cause of an event. Bulman and Wortman (1977) found that patients were more likely to blame themselves if they believed that they could have avoided the accident. Alternatively, this phenomenon could be explained by saying that if patients believed that they could have controlled the situation but did not, they were likely to assign an internal cause. This dimension was examined in detail in an earlier section.

Intentionality is the fourth dimension to be explored. This dimension refers to the degree to which an individual made a deliberate decision to act in such a way as to intend the observed outcome.

The global dimension is the last attributional dimension to be discussed. This dimension relates to the number and variety of activities and the outcomes affected. Global attributions influence a wide variety while specific attributions concentrate on immediate situations.

Attributions have at least two characteristics that are important to health educators: their perseverance and openness to error. Attributions appear to be remarkably stable over time. For example, Rudy (1980), in her study of MI patients, discovered that there was a high stability of causality over time once it had been established in the convalescent phase.

Attributions are also subject to error (Kelley, 1967). It is possible to hypothesize a number of factors that could contribute to attributional error. Most of those factors are similar to those listed as influencing the attribution process. For example, knowledge that the individual gathers and uses may be incorrect. The person's attitudes, values, assumptions, and expectations may also contribute to an erroneous attribution by eliminating correct but personally unacceptable attributions. Lastly, the individual's repertoire of labels may be limited and therefore may not include the correct one.

It is important to recognize the cumulative effect of these two characteristics. Attributions may be erroneous, a significant problem. This problem is compounded if the characteristic of perseverance is considered. Perseverance or stability implies that it would be quite difficult to correct erroneous attributions. Therefore if an individual has incorrectly attributed a cause to an event, the attribution will be influential despite attempts to correct it.

Attribution of causality or the cause ascribed to a health problem can be very influential in the individual's selection of health behaviors. The study of attributions could be described as being in an infancy stage, especially in health contexts. Preliminary information, however, indicates that health care providers would be supported in pursuing causality with the patients whom they are assisting to make changes in their health behaviors. Obviously there are other factors influencing the compliance of individuals, including patient intentions.

PATIENT INTENTIONS

PATIENT: Thanks for bringing me to the doctor. I just don't think I could have driven my car today. My back still hurts so much. The doctor said I need to swim at least three or four times a week and to take it easy the rest of the time. She said the swimming will make my back muscles stronger.

FRIEND: That's what she said the last time you saw her, wasn't it?

PATIENT: Yes. You know my husband has been nagging me to go swimming but I just haven't gotten there.

FRIEND: Do you intend to go this time? The pool is only a mile or so from your house. I could drive you sometimes.

PATIENT: No, not really. Maybe if I rest more it will help my back.

On emerging from the doctor's office, this patient has no *intention* of following at least one aspect of her doctor's recommendations. She seems to have knowledge about the regimen and why it has been prescribed. The support and encouragement of family and friends are evidently available, as well. Nonetheless, she will probably not follow the recommendation to swim three or four times a week. This noncompliance could be predicted in a relatively direct fashion by gathering information about the patient's intentions.

Intentions are the immediate determinants of behaviors, according to the theory of reasoned action proposed by Ajzen and Fishbein (1980). This theory explores the relationships among behaviors, beliefs, attitudes, and intentions. It is yet another example of the value-expectancy models and is therefore in the same category as the Health Belief Model and locus of control. The components of this theory and their relationship are shown in Figure 3–5.

Ultimately intentions are a function of an individual's beliefs. Those beliefs are focused on two issues. First, individuals' beliefs that a behavior will produce the expected outcome and their evaluations of those outcomes are called *behavioral beliefs*. Second, *normative beliefs* focus on what individuals perceive important others believe should be done about performing or not performing the behaviors. Normative beliefs involve the influence of family, friends, or others on the performance of a behavior *from the individuals' perspectives*. This may or may not actually reflect what others believe the individual should do.

Beliefs do not have a direct effect on behaviors but one that is mediated by attitudes. As Figure 3–5 illustrates, the effect of behavioral and normative beliefs on behaviors is mediated by the *attitude toward the behavior* and the *subjective norm*. The attitude toward the behavior reflects the individual's evaluation of performing the behavior; i.e., is it good or bad to undertake action X? The subjective norm is the "person's perception of the social pressures put on him to perform or not perform the behavior in question" (Ajzen & Fishbein, 1980, p. 6). It is reasonable to assume, according to the theory, that individuals will intend to perform behaviors if the attitudes toward the behavior and the subjective norms favor the behaviors.

One other element influences intention formation. The effects of the subjective norm and the attitude toward the behavior are not always equal. In some cases, the influence of others (i.e., the subjective norm) is greater than the individual's attitude toward the behavior. The reverse may be true in other situations. In the conversation recorded earlier, the patient's attitude toward the behavior seemed more influential than the subjective norms in her decision regarding swimming. The relative importance to the individual of the subjective norm and the attitude toward the behavior must be considered as illustrated in Figure 3–5.

Is the relationship between intentions and behaviors always a direct one? Obviously it is not. Everyone can recall situations in which good intentions were never translated into action. There are factors that can influence the relationship between behaviors and intentions. If those factors are taken into account, the predictive value of intentions is more secure. The primary factor is the time interval between the point at which an individual's intentions are elicited and when the behavior is expected. As that interval widens, the predictive ability of intentions weakens. For example, one response is elicited if a woman is asked if she intends to perform a self-breast examination by the end of the week. Her response may be quite different if she is asked whether she intends to do a self-breast examination in six months.

A prolonged interval between the statement of intention and the behavior opens the possibility of exposure of the individual to new information. If, for example, a

Figure 3–5 Intentions: Their Precedents and Consequences

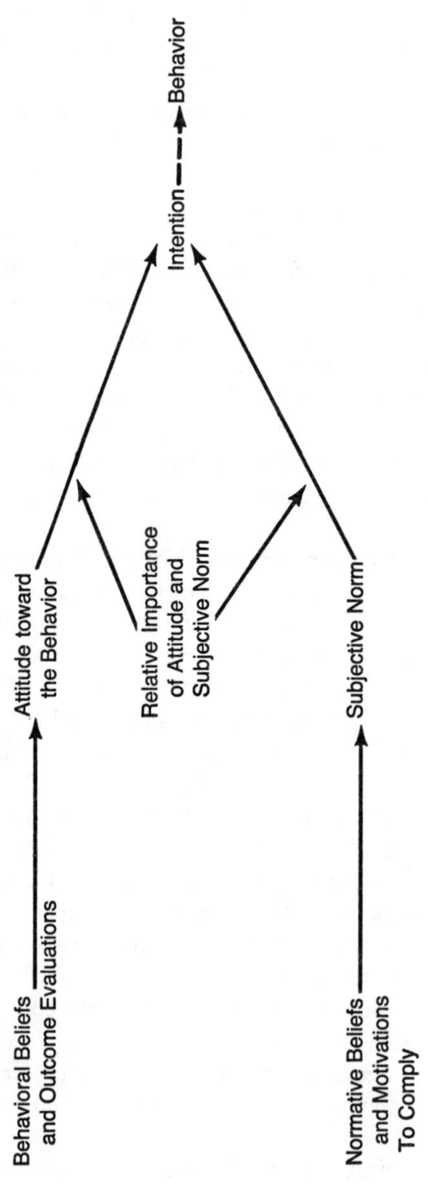

Source: Understanding Attitudes and Predicting Social Behavior (p. 100) by I. Ajzen and M. Fishbein, 1980. Englewood Cliffs, NJ: Prentice-Hall, Inc.

woman who had indicated that she did not intend to do self-breast examinations learns of a close friend's breast cancer, she might have a different intention.

Other factors can influence the behavior-intention relationship. In addition to time and additional knowledge, Jaccard (1975) lists several others. He includes the number of steps involved in the behavior (as that number increases, correspondence decreases), as well as the individual's memory, ability, and habits. Likewise, issues in measuring the intention and behavior can affect the relationship. Measurement problems can have a significant effect on the study of intentions and behaviors. The intentions measured must correspond precisely to the expected behaviors. For example, when attempting to predict whether an individual will stop smoking cigarettes at home this week, the measurement of intentions should also specify when smoking will stop, what type of smoking will cease (cigars, pipe, cigarettes), and where smoking will no longer take place (at home, at work, on social occasions) to maximize their predictive capacity.

Ajzen and Fishbein (1980) suggest another factor that will influence the relationship between intentions and behaviors. They propose that individuals with previous experience are more likely to have stable intentions, possibly because they have more realistic expectations.

Intentions are not considered predictors of outcomes. Factors other than an individual's behaviors can affect outcomes. Behavior and outcomes cannot be equated.

There is a paucity of research about the theory of reasoned action in the health behavior context. It was studied in relation to post–myocardial infarction patients by Miller, Johnson, Garrett, Wickoff, and McMahon (1982). One part of their study examined the patient's intentions, subjective norms, and compliance with prescribed dietary exercise, stress modification, medication, and smoking behaviors. They found a significant relationship between intentions and adherence when dietary behavior was studied ($p <.001$). A significant relationship was not demonstrated when intentions and the other behaviors were studied. A significant relationship between normative beliefs (perceptions of what others think the individual should do) and adherence to medication prescriptions was found ($p <.01$). Likewise, the prescribed influence of others significantly influenced diet ($p <.05$), exercise ($p <.001$), and stress modification ($p <.001$ at 6 months). While their findings did not absolutely support each component of the theory, future study is encouraged. In addition, their findings concerning the relationship between the prescribed influence of others and the individuals' intentions is an important one. Of note is their observation that "patients consistently perceived family members' expectations to be higher than their own intentions or behavior . . . (and) that the patient's perception of his family members' expectations was more closely related to patient behavior than the patient's own intentions" (p. 338).

In another study, weight loss was examined from the perspective of the theory of reasoned action. Sejwacz, Ajzen, and Fishbein (1980) found that actual dieting behavior and increasing physical activity were related to the individual's intentions to perform each behavior. In turn, the amount of weight lost was partly related to the extent to which those activities were performed. In the course of the study, intentions to perform specific as well as general weight loss activities were examined. The researchers found that the specific activity intentions (i.e., to avoid snacking, to walk instead of drive, etc.) had more predictive value.

What value does the study of intentions, encompassed by the theory of reasoned action, have for health educators? As in other approaches to understanding and predicting health behaviors, there is considerable value to this theory. It emphasizes the individual's perceptions, an important factor in subsequent activities. Thus what the person perceives is critical to the situation, and perceptions of the health educator assume a lesser role. The influences of two key ingredients—individual beliefs and perceptions of social pressures—are included in the study of intentions. There is also an emphasis on the individual behaviors included in the therapeutic regimen rather than on the regimen as a whole. That emphasis challenges educators to evaluate each aspect of the therapeutic regimen.

The study of intentions provides an assessment mechanism for use in predicting whether patients will comply with prescribed regimens. As Jaccard (1975) observes:

> A person will probably perform a behavior if he or she *intends* to perform the behavior and probably will not perform the behavior if he or she intends not to perform it. If one wishes to forecast an individual's behavior, probably the simplest and most efficient way of doing so is to ask the individual if he or she *intends* to perform the behavior in question. (p. 153)

Thus, it may be helpful for health educators to ask if the patient intends to perform the behaviors prescribed in the therapeutic regimen. Given that the relationship between intentions and behaviors weakens as the time interval lengthens, it is probably reasonable to assume that an individual's intentions should be reassessed during each contact, especially in an outpatient setting.

Other factors influencing patient compliance with therapeutic regimens are investigated in the next section.

FACTORS RELATED TO THE ILLNESS ITSELF

The illness and its features can greatly influence rates of compliance. Two major factors are to be considered when the effect of the illness is examined. One factor concerns the presence or absence of symptoms, and the other involves the characteristics of the illness.

The experience of symptoms is an overwhelming factor influencing the decision to seek care. Kirscht and Rosenstock (1980) noted that "when people are ill the presence of symptoms forms a focal event for reacting to advice. . . . While symptom occurrence is not a sufficient condition for adherence it is a factor in personal readiness to act on medical advice" (p. 194). Additionally, Becker and Maiman (1980) observed that "the situation of non-compliance worsens markedly where the patients are symptom free" (p. 113). Symptom occurrence, however, does not necessarily predict how care is sought or whether the patient eventually complies with resulting advice.

Symptoms vary widely in their usefulness in predicting compliance with therapeutic regimens. Symptoms differ from situation to situation, making them difficult to evaluate. Quite often symptoms are transient, and this further confuses individuals as they attempt to interpret their significance and make decisions about seeking care. Then, too, individuals differ in their responses to the experience of symptoms. Some of the variation may be explained by culture, which can influence the patient's willingness to discuss symptoms or to pursue relief from symptoms.

Symptoms are also used by patients to evaluate the effectiveness of treatment regimens. For example, Gutmann and his colleagues (1979) found that 92 percent of their 50 patients maintained that they could monitor their blood pressure elevations even though they agreed that most people could not. Sixty-eight percent of the patients treated for hypertension perceived their medication as affecting the sign or symptom that they were using as a monitor. All but one of these patients were taking their medications as prescribed or reported infrequent missed doses and they were more likely to be under better blood pressure control. However, Hulka and her colleagues (1976) did not find a relationship between the duration of the disease or its severity and drug errors. They studied errors of omission, commission, and scheduling.

Sometimes symptom relief provides an incentive for the patient to adhere to the prescribed regimen. Such was the case of Mrs. Walker, a 62-year-old patient with rheumatoid arthritis. Initially she did not carry out medication or physical therapy prescriptions. As her condition progressed, Mrs. Walker needed hospitalization. During the hospitalization her symptoms were alleviated through medication and prescribed exercises. She also received extensive education about her condition and its treatment. Following the hospitalization, Mrs. Walker followed her regimen faithfully in an effort to remain symptom free.

Symptom relief can have the opposite effect. A classic example centers on Judy, a 19-year-old patient who presented in the emergency clinic with a urinary tract infection. She was prescribed a 10-day medication regimen. However, because her symptoms disappeared after 6 days, Judy independently discontinued her medications. Unfortunately she suffered a relapse and required prolonged treatment to obliterate the infection.

Specific characteristics of the illness may also have an impact on compliance levels. Significant characteristics include

- How severe is the illness? This was highlighted by Watts (1966), who found a consistently high correlation between the severity of illness and the treatment obtained.
- What is the stage of the illness? Is the patient newly diagnosed or chronically ill? Has this patient sought advice for health maintenance? Does the patient believe self to be at risk for developing a disease or condition and therefore requested information and advice? The patient's current stage of health or illness will influence compliance, and each stage presents different health education needs. Some studies have demonstrated that newly diagnosed patients are more likely to comply with recommended regimens. Likewise, Sackett (1978) found that medication compliance diminished markedly with the passage of time. The stage of illness or wellness is an important consideration for patient educators as they assess the patient's need for education.
- How visible is the illness to others? Patients whose symptomatology is not readily detected by others do not reap the rewards of being ill, only the responsibilities. They must, therefore, be able to sustain their actions over long periods without consistent support, a difficult and sometimes impossible task. "Invisible" illnesses are extremely common; hypertension and diabetes are two ready examples.
- Has the patient had previous experience with this illness or other illnesses? Previous experience with an illness will sometimes arm patients with the knowledge that they need to interpret their symptoms more accurately. This may, in turn, contribute to their willingness and ability to comply with subsequent prescribed regimens. For example, Becker, Drachman, and Kirscht (1974) found that experience with ear infections (either in the currently ill child or others) predicted compliance with the prescribed medications.

The presence of symptoms and various characteristics of the illness can have a profound impact on the patient's level of compliance. They are factors well worth assessing when planning patient education strategies.

FACTORS RELATED TO THE PRESCRIBED REGIMEN

One of the most important factors influencing patient compliance is the treatment plan prescribed. Some researchers and practitioners even cite this factor as the most critical of all potential impediments or enhancers of compliance. Therefore as strategies for patient education are planned, one of the key steps is to examine the regimen that the patient has been asked to implement.

The first step in evaluating the regimen is to list each activity associated with the patient's treatment plan and each goal developed. This process is one phase in the overall process of conducting an educationally focused patient assessment, a topic discussed in detail in the next section. All prescribed behaviors should be included, whether they are being added, deleted, or modified. At this point the treatment regimen can be critically examined.

The ultimate goal of this process is to arrive at a treatment plan that is likely to succeed and that will effectively treat the problem at hand. Answers to the questions generated by the criteria may necessitate a change in treatment plan or some compromise for both parties. Ultimately, however, the plan may be more palatable for the patient and thus more successful.

There are several criteria involved in evaluating a treatment regimen. Those criteria include the following:

- effectiveness
- complexity
- cost
- side effects
- convenience
- duration
- available support and supervision
- behavior change required
- patient perceptions
- results

These criteria are useful to both practitioners and patients. In fact, patients usually apply most of these criteria, either instinctively or deliberately, when determining whether to carry out prescribed behavior changes.

Each criterion generates a series of specific questions that can be used to evaluate the regimen. Some questions generated by the criteria and subsequent observations are outlined in the following section.

Effectiveness. An important criterion is whether the treatment plan will accomplish the desired goals. There is also concern about whether alternative approaches to the condition or problem exist and if they would be as effective. The question evoked by this criterion, then, is whether the proposed treatment plan or its alternatives will be effective in dealing with the problem.

Complexity. There is support for the hypothesis that as the number of treatments involved in a regimen increases, the likelihood of compliance diminishes. Practitioners acknowledge this as a factor in that 51 percent of the respondents to the authors' survey indicated that noncompliance can be caused by the complexity of the regimen. Becker and Maiman (1980) noted that patient compliance is likely to be enhanced when changes are made in the regimen that decrease its complexity, duration, alterations in life style, inconvenience, or cost. In a similar manner, errors of omission and commission have been noted to increase with increasing numbers of components in the regimen. This is especially true when increasing numbers of drugs are prescribed (Falvo et al., 1980; Sackett, 1978; Hulka, Kupper, Cassel, Efird, & Burdette, 1975; Hulka et al., 1976; Marston, 1970).

The complexity of the regimen becomes evident when the practitioner reviews the written list of the treatment plan components, the process suggested earlier as the first step in evaluating the regimen. The questions generated by this criterion include: How many components are involved in the treatment program for this patient? Are all the components necessary? Are some components more important than others? Could any be deleted or delayed? How complex are the individual components?

Cost. The cost of a therapeutic regimen will greatly influence a patient's compliance. This was recognized by the practitioners responding to the authors' survey. Eighty-two percent believed that the expense of the regimen (money, time, or effort) was associated with patient noncompliance. The Health Belief Model incorporates the concept of perceived barriers to action, and cost is often such a barrier for patients. A staff nurse whose husband became ill provides an example of how cost could influence compliance. When this couple had the medication prescription filled, the total cost was $65 for a 7-day regimen. She commented: "That definitely could influence compliance. However, we decided that he was worth it and that we could afford to pay this. Others may need to make different choices." Health educators should develop a habit of calculating how much various treatment plans will cost the patient. This is especially valuable for those treatments frequently prescribed by the practitioner. Then an assessment of how much of the cost will be paid by the patient's insurance carrier or other third party agencies should be made. The next question is whether the patient can and will handle the remaining expenses.

The assessment of cost does not rest exclusively with expenses directly involved in hospitalization, clinic visits, or prescriptions. What other costs will the patient incur? Time expenditure, loss of time or pay from work, necessity to pay a babysitter, the costs of necessary home modifications (e.g., ramps or lowered sinks) are expenses that the patient will use to evaluate whether the treatment plan is affordable.

An example of this type of situation involved Cheryl, a 5-year-old child hospitalized for high blood levels of lead. She had been hospitalized numerous times for the same problem. Her parents were aware that the paint used in their old house was probably filled with lead and that Cheryl was eating paint chips. However, it was not financially feasible for them to move or to repaint the house. As a result, Cheryl's health problems continued.

Side Effects. Many therapeutic regimens produce side effects that are very uncomfortable for the patient. In some cases, the side effects make the patient feel worse than the actual disease for which the treatment was prescribed. Treatment for hypertension is one example in that antihypertensive medications may produce side effects that are much more unpleasant than the disease itself. The occurrence of side effects is significant because they may lead to noncompliance. For example, Nelson and his colleagues (1980) found that 69% of the patients who reported that their antihypertensive medications had given them side effects were noncompliant. Kirscht and Rosenstock (1977) also noted that patients who experienced side effects had a tendency not to take all their prescribed medications.

Therefore, when the treatment regimen is evaluated in terms of the side effects that it will produce, the practitioner needs to ask if there is a way to minimize or counteract the expected side effects. In any case, it is critical that the patient be advised of the likelihood of side effects and what can be done if they occur. Providing the patient with this information facilitates coping and cooperation with the treatment plan. If patients are unaware that side effects are expected, they may decide to discontinue the medication or treatment because they fear that the reaction is untoward.

Convenience. Treatment plans that fit smoothly into the patient's usual life style have a greater likelihood of success than those which are extremely disruptive. Ferguson and Bole (1979) theorized that their arthritic patients were more likely to take aspirin than exercise or use splints because aspirin-taking required less effort. Likewise, Nelson and his colleagues (1980) found that "respondents who indicated hypertension had disrupted their life styles tended to be poor compliers" (p. 509). Kirscht and Rosenstock (1977) found that patients who reported little or no difficulty in following the doctor's advice also tended to report compliance with the prescribed regimen. In a similar fashion, Procci (1978), in a study of hemodialysis patients, reported that patients who continued employment throughout their dialysis program were more likely to be good compliers. Finally, in another study of hemodialysis patients, Kirilloff (1981) found that 50 percent of the noncompliant patients reported difficulty in adapting the treatments to their previous life style. Therefore it is useful to ask what impact the plan will have on the patient's ability to carry out the usual way of life and then determine what steps will minimize that effect as much as possible.

Duration. There is also support for the hypothesis that compliance tends to diminish over time. For example, Sackett (1978) found that medication compliance diminished markedly with the passage of time. Cummings and his colleagues (1982) found that patients on dialysis for lengthy periods tended to be poor compliers, as did Bollin and Hart. As a result, the length of time that the patient will be required to fulfill the treatment regimen becomes a critical element in assessing the impact of the regimen. The practitioner needs to consider the minimum amount of time that the patient will need to comply as well as the maximum time. Another aspect of this criterion is to determine whether the time frame can be shortened with reasonable safety and continued effectiveness.

The patients' own beliefs about how long the regimen must last will also influence health behaviors. Patient estimates of the time frame may vary considerably from those of the prescriber. Nelson and his colleagues (1980) found that noncompliance was related to the belief that treatment of hypertension need not be lifelong. This implies that patients and prescribers need to discuss the length of time that the treatment program will be needed. Likewise, it is important to ask patients how long they expect to be on a particular program.

Available Support and Supervision. This criterion is especially important when treatment plans of long duration are contemplated. As an example, Nelson and his colleagues (1980) found that the patient's lack of someone to share problems with was one variable related to noncompliance.

Support stems from many resources. Family, friends, and health care providers are just a few possible sources. The assessment of the regimen should include information about whether supports are available to the patient and if they are likely to be used. At times, support may be available, but the patient may be unable or unwilling to utilize it. This was the case of Mr. T., a 34-year-old Mexican-American patient who was a quadriplegic as a result of a cervical injury. On discharge Mr. T. needed assistance with bladder and bowel care. He and his family could not afford home nursing care and his wife became his caregiver. However, he was reluctant to use this assistance because it conflicted with his macho self-image. He also refused assistance from male relatives because it made him more aware of "no longer being a man," and he did not want them to see the extent of his disability. Consequently he repeatedly returned to the hospital with bladder complications.

It is equally important to determine which family member will be providing the patient's care at home. This was illustrated by the case of Christopher, a 3½-year-old boy with cystic fibrosis. Christopher experienced a number of admissions for his disease and presented with increased respiratory distress and congestion on each admission. The parents emphasized that they carried out each aspect of the treatment plan, including medications and postural drainage. However, Christopher did not improve and in fact periodically became very ill. One afternoon Christopher's father offered to do the scheduled postural drainage. The nurse accepted the offer and used the opportunity to observe his technique. While observing the treatment, she realized that if this were the way in which the treatment had been administered at home, it had not been done correctly. On further investigation the nurse discovered that Christopher's mother received extensive training in postural drainage during his newborn and infancy admissions. However, his father was doing all his postural drainage treatments at home.

Within limits, compliance increases with supervision. As Blackwell (1973) noted, "Those who are most closely supervised in the hospital or at home are most likely to comply" (p. 251). Therefore, the necessity for and availability of intermittent supervision are a factor to be considered when evaluating the treatment program. If supports are not readily available, how can such support systems be developed?

Behavior Change Required. Is the patient being asked to omit a behavior, modify a behavior, or add a behavior? Patients tend to be more successful at adding behaviors than omitting or modifying them (Ozuna, 1981). This was confirmed by the practitioners responding to the authors' survey. Seventy-six percent indicated that it is more difficult for patients to change or delete behaviors than to add behaviors. The behaviors in each treatment program need to be evaluated carefully to determine what kind of change is being prescribed.

Patient Perceptions. Most patients have their own ideas and beliefs about the regimens prescribed and about their state of health. Some parts of the prescription are perceived as easily managed or important and others seen as difficult or unimportant. To a large extent, the patient's perceptions determine the willingness to undertake recommended actions and then actually to carry them out. A mechanism to elicit patients' perceptions of their health problems and the preferred course of action becomes essential.

For patients who are alert, oriented, and able to follow directions, consider having them complete the health problem self-assessment tool independently (Exhibit 3–4). The patient should be asked to complete one line before moving on to the next. The completed self-assessment can then be reviewed with the patient and points of confusion clarified. If the patient is unable to complete such an assessment independently, the practitioner can use the tool as a guide for eliciting information about the patient's perceptions of the problem. The important task is to determine, in some way, the *patient's* perceptions of the health problems and the recommended regimen.

Results. What sort of results can the patient expect if the therapeutic regimen is followed faithfully? How soon should the results become evident? Will the results be visible or otherwise noticeable? Will the patient improve, be maintained at the current status, or continue to deteriorate? What does the patient think will and should happen? Often the expectations of the patient and the practitioner differ, sometimes widely. The patient needs to have a clear picture of the expected results of various activities. Many of the regimens prescribed for patients lack feedback or

Exhibit 3–4 Health Problem Self-Assessment

Date ____________		Patient ____________ Primary Physician ____________ Primary Nurse ____________	
I think my health problems are or could be	*I will know when the problem is better when I*	*Some of the things that will help me get better or avoid a health problem are*	*Things that may get in my way are*

observable results. It is very difficult to continue with an action if progress is not forthcoming. The hypertensive, for example, who restricts salt and faithfully adheres to prescribed medication schedules will not necessarily observe results.

It is especially discouraging to patients and their families when results are not evident despite an investment of limited resources. Beth, an 11-month-old girl with transposition of the great vessels, presents a typical situation. Beth's parents have very limited financial resources. Her cardiac status is fragile, and Beth frequently develops congestive heart failure despite medication. Her parents stopped giving Beth digoxin because "it was so expensive and it didn't work anyway." As a result, Beth presented in the emergency room with severe congestive heart failure.

A related question, then, is to determine if there is any way that the consequences of behaviors can be made more observable. Referring to the hypertensive patient, will learning how to take blood pressure make the condition more concrete? Or are there other ways that the outcomes of the therapeutic regimen can become visible?

EDUCATIONALLY FOCUSED PATIENT ASSESSMENTS

All health practitioners utilize a defined, standardized approach to the care of patients. This approach includes several phases, notably, gathering information, making a diagnosis (or defining the problem), establishing goals (or desired outcomes), developing and implementing interventions, evaluating the results and effectiveness of the interventions, and, finally, revising any of the activities of the previous phases if necessary. This process is also beneficial in the course of patient education. Indeed, Jenkins (1979) notes that "dealing with disorders of health related behaviors is much like dealing with other health disorders in that they all need an appropriate diagnostic workup, treatment planning and evaluation of the intervention" (p. 11).

The goal of assessing and diagnosing individuals' responses to therapeutic regimens is to identify areas in which they will need support and assistance. In addition, the health educator is attempting to identify those patients for whom compliance with the prescribed regimen will be difficult or improbable. When this information is obtained, it may be possible to develop specific strategies to support patients in their efforts to comply.

This process will lead the practitioner toward establishing a diagnosis regarding health behaviors. This is an important phase of the patient education process. Indeed, *noncompliance* and *knowledge deficit* were two nursing diagnoses accepted at the Fourth (1980) Conference on Nursing Diagnosis (Gordon, 1982, p. 320).

Many elements should be incorporated in an educationally focused patient assessment. The first categories of information usually obtained deal with the knowledge and skills that the patient must have to carry out the regimen. This assessment, however, must extend beyond the category of educational needs to include a review of factors that will interfere with or enhance the learning and compliance processes for the individual. Bartlett (1982) proposed that the following classifications be included in the behavioral diagnosis format: individual factors (such as knowledge, attitudes, and beliefs), social factors, environmental factors, and information about the therapeutic regimen. Demographic factors were previously discussed as having little or no consistent effect on patient compliance. However, it is useful to include such information in an educational assessment in order to provide a more complete picture of the individual and because it may influence the teaching strategies selected.

Patient perceptions of all aspects of the diagnosed problem or regimen should also be incorporated. This would include perceptions of susceptibility, barriers to the regimen's activities, causes of the problem, as well as the other psychosocial factors discussed earlier in this chapter. A critical examination of the regimen (its complexity, duration, etc.) is another element in a comprehensive assessment. Those factors that may enhance the patient's ability to follow the regimen should be included in the assessment process.

A sample education-focused assessment tool is included in Exhibit 3–5. Each practitioner will probably develop a format or method of proceeding that meets the individual's needs. Others may adapt a different format to respond to the need of their specific populations of patients or situations.

Diagnosing issues in compliance with prescribed regimens is a process that cannot be rushed. It depends, in part, on the relationship developed between the patient and the practitioner. An educational assessment will probably not be completed in the first encounter with the patient. Rather, the process will extend over time. The earlier observation that patient compliance is not consistent over time indicates the need to reassess its status on a frequent, regular basis.

For practitioners who deal with fairly consistent diagnostic groups of patients, it may be helpful to maintain updated information about commonly used treatment elements. For example, practitioners working with stoma patients will want to maintain current information about the cost of the equipment involved in their care. In this way, the practitioners will be able to discuss realistically the costs involved in their patients' care and to recognize more readily when this is likely to be a problem.

The actual process of eliciting information from patients and their families is that used in any form of patient interview. Practitioners who need a review of these techniques are referred to one of the many excellent books or articles on interviewing. As in other contexts, interviews for patient education purposes should incorporate the use of open-ended questions where the patients can elaborate on the subject at hand. It may be less threatening to patients to approach the sensitive topic of compliance with an acknowledgment that other patients have reported difficulties with particular aspects of their regimen. This allows the practitioner to ask patients if they anticipate problems with any of the prescribed activities. For example, the cardiac patient may be approached regarding a planned exercise routine by noting that "a number of patients have told me that they have trouble fitting their exercises into their usual daily activities. Do you think that will be a problem for you?"

Timing is another important consideration. Most patients need time to recover from the stress of learning about their new condition or treatment plan before discussing their reactions to it or the feasibility of complying with the plan. A telephone call a few days after the treatment plan has been initially discussed may be the opportune time to determine aspects of the plan that are problematic for the patient. Another approach may be to schedule a follow-up appointment with the patient within a short time after initiating the treatment plan. Then, too, emphasiz-

Exhibit 3–5 Education-Focused Patient Assessment

DEMOGRAPHIC DATA

Patient name ______________________

Age ______ Sex ______ Marital status ________ Religion ______________

Number and ages of children ______________________

Educational background ______________________

DIAGNOSIS-RELATED DATA

Health Problem List and Priority	
Patient's Description	Nurse's Description
1. ______________	1. ______________
2. ______________	2. ______________
3. ______________	3. ______________
4. ______________	4. ______________
5. ______________	5. ______________

Which of the problems listed are acute or newly diagnosed? ______________
______________ Chronic? ______________
____

What knowledge does the patient currently have about these problems (symptoms, cause, treatment, etc.)? ______________
____
____

List symptomatology involved. ______________
____

How have these problems affected the patient's life style (mobility, ADL, diet, job, etc.)?
____
____

What has the patient gained by being ill (attention, etc.)? ______________
____
____
____

What aspects of these health problems are visible to others? ______________
____

Exhibit 3–5 continued

Complications expected by the patient? ______________________________

____

______________ by the nurse? ______________________________

____

How serious does the patient believe the condition to be? ______________

____

____

PATIENT SUPPORT SYSTEMS

What medical or nursing support is available to the patient? ______________

____

______________________________ Is the patient willing or able to use that support? (Explain.) ______________________________

____

____

Which of the patient's family and friends can the patient count on for support and assistance with these problems? ______________________________

____

____

What do the patient's family and friends think should be done about the identified health problems? ______________________________

____

____

REGIMEN-RELATED DATA

Regimen Component	*Add/Modify/ Delete Behavior*	*Duration*
______________	______________	______________
______________	______________	______________
______________	______________	______________
______________	______________	______________
______________	______________	______________
______________	______________	______________
______________	______________	______________

What does the patient think needs to be done about the problems identified? ______________

____

____

Exhibit 3–5 continued

What alternatives exist for the proposed treatment plan? ____________________

____

____

Describe Anticipated Results

Patient	*Nurse*
____________________	____________________
____________________	____________________
____________________	____________________
____________________	____________________
____________________	____________________

When Will Results Be Apparent?

Patient	*Nurse*
____________________	____________________
____________________	____________________

What will the cost of the regimen be to the patient in terms of money, time, and other factors?

____

____

What will make it difficult for the patient to fulfill the components of the regimen? ________

____

____________________ What can be done to facilitate the treatment plan?

____

____

Does the patient have the necessary physical skills and coordination to do the tasks required by the regimen? (Explain.) ____________________

____

____

PSYCHOSOCIAL VARIABLES

Does the patient think he can affect the quality of his health or is good health a matter of luck?

____

Does the patient prefer to control what is happening to him or would he rather leave it to his nurse or doctor? ____________________

____

Exhibit 3–5 continued

EDUCATIONAL STRATEGY CONSIDERATIONS

Has the patient been successful in complying with treatment regimens in the past? ________
________ Describe positive or negative experiences. ________

What experiences has the patient had with health care? ________

Does the patient know anyone who has this or a similar problem? ________
Describe. ________

Does the regimen involve knowledge or skills similar to those already possessed by the patient? (Describe.) ________

What values are important to the patient? ________

Does the patient intend to follow the therapeutic regimen? ________

ADDITIONAL RELEVANT INFORMATION ________

____
Signature and Title

ing to the patient that telephone calls with questions or problems would be welcome, can be helpful. Specific times when calls are more convenient for the practitioner may reassure the patient that a busy schedule is not being interrupted.

Although the amount of information involved in an educationally focused assessment seems extreme, much of it is obtained during the usual history and physical assessment of the patient. This information, then, is already available for inclusion in the educational assessment. The value of transferring the information to the educational assessment lies in establishing the proper context. In other words, all the factors involved in the patient's education can be examined simultaneously, and their interrelationships become more apparent.

Those who practice in settings where ongoing patient contact does not occur, such as in emergency rooms or ambulatory surgical centers, will need to develop special skills, systems, and techniques for assessing and monitoring patient compliance with recommended treatments. Techniques that allow the alert patient to complete portions of the assessment may be helpful in saving practitioners time and allowing them to focus on intervention strategies. Follow-up techniques, such as those outlined earlier, may also facilitate patient compliance after discharge from the area. Establishing a routine or abbreviated format for assessing the educational needs and influences of patients in these areas contributes greatly to understanding and identifying patients for whom compliance with therapeutic regimens will be difficult.

In summary, an educationally focused patient assessment process can contribute to the success of patient educators' activities. As Bartlett (1982) observed:

> Although we have no proof that arriving at a correct behavioral diagnosis will improve the effectiveness of patient education, it seems plausible that educational efforts directed at the influences of behavior will be more effective than those that aim solely at teaching the patient the facts of the disease and the regimen. Further research is needed to apply the behavioral diagnosis approach to a wider range of medical and behavioral problems, to identify the most effective and practical methods of performing a behavioral diagnosis and to determine the extent to which the findings from one patient can be generalized to other patients with similar problems. (pp. 33–34)

SUMMARY

The issue of patient compliance is complex. Many elements of compliance have emotional overtones for the health care provider as well as for the patient. In addition, the direct and indirect expenses associated with noncompliance can be considerable.

Increasingly the responsibility for health care is being redistributed to the patient. Health care providers are assuming a more indirect, supervisory role in many cases. As a result, patients are managing highly complex self-care situations. Indeed, patients often carry out procedures such as intravenous therapy or intermittent urinary catheterization that would have necessitated prolonged hospitalization in previous times. Sometimes self-care must take place despite nonsupportive social environments. The consequences of noncompliance may be extremely detrimental to the patient's overall well-being.

The effects of noncompliance extend well beyond the individual patient. The circle of family and friends is likely to be affected. Availability of health care services can be compromised if noncompliance results in recidivism. Costs associated with care will increase, adding to the financial burdens of individuals as well as society or the nation at large.

Many factors can influence patient compliance levels. Those factors may be internal to individuals and their support systems; they may involve the relationship developed with health care providers or be related to the illness or prescribed regimen. Ultimately the solution is likely to involve all those categories of factors, some more influential at various times than at others.

The issue of compliance also offers a unique opportunity to health care providers to plan and implement creative, supportive strategies. This is simultaneously one of the most creative, yet demanding aspects of health care practice.

Patient education has largely relied on a didactic, explanatory approach. Recognition of potential or actual cases of noncompliance has primarily been the result of the intuitive sense of the practitioner. As patients assume responsibility for increasingly complex self-care, however, practitioners must become more adept at identifying and effectively supporting those who are at risk for compliance difficulties. That skill involves knowledge about factors influencing compliance, developing relationships with patients, interviewing and assessing, and teaching strategies. This chapter has provided information about factors influencing compliance. Other chapters review additional information about the process of patient education.

Additional research is needed to support theories such as the Health Belief Model or attribution theory. Patient educators can make a contribution by approaching the teaching process with a sense of inquiry and by conducting research. In addition, they can apply research findings in their practice.

Patients face an enormous task in coping with therapeutic regimens. The education process is one means of supporting patients in this endeavor, especially when it is founded on an understanding of compliance issues.

REFERENCES

Ajzen, I., & Fishbein, M. (1980). *Understanding attitudes and predicting social behavior*. Englewood Cliffs, NJ: Prentice-Hall, Inc.

Andreoli, K.G. (1981). Self-concepts and health beliefs in compliant and noncompliant hypertensive patients. *Nursing Research 30*(6), 323–328.

Baric, L. (1969). Recognition of the "at risk" role: A means to influence health behavior. *International Journal of Health Education 12*(1), 24–34.

Bartlett, E. (1982). Behavioral diagnosis: A practical approach to patient education. *Patient Counselling and Health Education 4*(1), 29–35.

Becker, M. (Ed.). (1974). *The health belief model and personal health behavior*. Thorofare, NJ: Charles B. Slack.

Becker, M., Drachman, R., & Kirscht, J. (1972). Motivations as predictors of health behavior. *Health Services Reports 89*(9), 852–862.

Becker, M., Drachman, R., & Kirscht, J. (1974). A new approach to explaining sick role behavior in low income populations. *American Journal of Public Health 64*(3), 205–216.

Becker, M., Drachman, R., & Kirscht, J. (1978). Predicting mothers' compliance with pediatric medical regimens. *Medical Care 81*(4), 843–854.

Becker, M., & Maiman, L. (1975). Sociobehavioral determinants of compliance with health and medical care recommendations. *Medical Care 13*(1), 10–24.

Becker, M., & Maiman, L. (1980). Strategies for enhancing patient compliance. *Journal of Community Health 6*(2), 113–135.

Blackwell, B. (1973). Drug therapy: Patient compliance. *New England Journal of Medicine 289*(5), 249–252.

Blackwell, B. (1978, Fall). Counselling and compliance. *Patient Counselling and Health Education 1*(2), 45–49.

Blaxter, M. (1983). The causes of disease: Women talking. *Social Science and Medicine 17*(2), 59–69.

Bollin, B.W., & Hart, L.K. (1982). The relationship of health belief motivations, health locus of control and health valuing to dietary compliance of hemodialysis patients. *AANNT Journal 9*(5), 41–47.

Bulman, R.J., & Wortman, C.G. (1977). Attribution of blame and coping in the "real world": Severe accident victims react to their lot. *Journal of Personality and Social Psychology 35*, 351–363.

Charney, E. (1975). Compliance and prescribance. *American Journal of Diseases of Children 129*(9), 1009–1010.

Dabbs, J.M., & Kirscht, J.P. (1978). "Internal control" and the taking of influenza shots. *Psychological Reports 28*, 959–962.

Davis, M. (1966). Variations in patients' compliance with doctors' orders: Analysis of consequence between survey responses and results of empirical investigations. *Journal of Medical Education 44*(11), 1037–1048.

Davis, M. (1968). Variations in patient's compliance with doctors' advice: An empirical analysis of patterns of communication. *American Journal of Public Health 58*(2), 274–288.

DiMatteo, M., Prince, L., & Taranta, A. (1979). Patient perceptions of physicians' behavior: Determinants of commitment to the therapeutic relationship. *Journal of Community Health 4*(4), 280–290.

Fabrega, H., Jr. (1973). Toward a model of illness behavior. *Health Care 1*(6), 470–484.

Falvo, D., Woehlke, P., & Deichmann, J. (1980). Relationship of physician behavior to patient compliance. *Patient Counselling and Health Education 3*(4), 185–188.

Ferguson, K., & Bole, G. (1979). Family support, health beliefs and therapeutic compliance in patients with rheumatoid arthritis. *Patient Counselling and Health Education*, 101–104.

Finnerty, F., Jr. (1981). Hypertension: Specially trained personnel can improve compliance. *Consultant 21*(3), 80–90.

Fuchs, V.R. (1974). *Who shall live?* New York: Basic Books.

Gillum, R., & Barsky, A. (1974). Diagnosis and management of patient noncompliance. *Journal of the American Medical Association 228*(12), 1563–1567.

Goldstein, A., & Reznikoff, M. (1971). Suicide in chronic hemodialysis patients from an external LOC framework. *American Journal of Psychiatry 129*(9), 1204–1207.

Goldstein, K. (1959). Health as value. In A. Maslow (Ed.), *New knowledge in human values*. New York: Harper & Row.

Gordon, M. (1982). *Nursing diagnosis: Process and application*. New York: McGraw-Hill Book Co.

Gutmann, M.C., Meyer, D., Leventhal, H., Gutmann, F.D., & Jackson, T. (1979, May). *Medical versus patient-oriented interviewing*. Paper presented at the national meeting, American Federation for Clinical Research, Washington, DC.

Hulka, B., Cassel, J.C., Kupper, L.L., & Burdette, J.A. (1976). Communication, compliance and concordance between physicians and patients with prescribed medications. *American Journal of Public Health 66*(9), 847–848.

Hulka, B., Kupper, L., Cassel, J., Efird, R., & Burdette, J. (1975). Medication use and misuse: Physician-patient discrepancies. *Journal of Chronic Diseases 28*(1), 7–21.

Jaccard, J. (1975). A theoretical analysis of selected factors important to education strategies. *Health Education Monographs 78*, 152–167.

Jenkins, C.D. (1979). An approach to the diagnosis and treatment of problems of health related behavior [supplement]. *International Journal of Health Behavior 22*(2), 1–24.

Kanouse, D.E. (1972). Language, labeling and attribution. In E. Jones, D. Kanouse, H. Kelley, R. Nisbett, S. Valins, & B. Weiner (Eds.), *Attribution: Perceiving the causes of behavior*. Morristown, NJ: General Learning Press.

Kelley, H.H. (1967). Attribution theory in social psychology. In D. Levine (Ed.), *Nebraska symposium on motivation*. Lincoln: University of Nebraska Press.

Kirilloff, L. (1981). Factors influencing the compliance of hemodialysis patients with their therapeutic regimen. *AANNT Journal 8*(4), 15–20.

Kirscht, J.P., & Rosenstock, I.M. (1977). Patient adherence to antihypertensive medical regimens. *Journal of Community Health 3*(2), 115–125.

Kirscht, J., & Rosenstock, I. (1980). Patients' problems in following recommendations of health experts. In G. Stone, F. Cohen, & N. Adler (Eds.), *Health psychology*. San Francisco: Jossey-Bass Pubs.

Lau, R. (1982). Origins of health locus of control beliefs. *Journal of Personality and Social Psychology 42*(2), 322–334.

Lau, R.R., & Hartman, K.A. (1983). Common sense representations of common illness. *Health Psychology 2*(2), 167–185.

Lefcourt, H. (1982). Locus of control: *Current trends in theory and research*. Hillsdale, NJ: Lawrence Erlbaum Associates.

Leventhal, H., & Hirschman, R.S. (1982). Social psychology and prevention. In G.S. Sanders & J. Suls (Eds.), *Social psychology of health and illness*. Hillsdale, NJ: PRODIST.

Ley, P. (1972). Primacy, rated importance and the recall of medical statements. *Journal of Health and Social Behavior 13*(3), 311–318.

MacDonald, A.P., Jr. (1970). I-E locus of control and the practice of birth control. *Psychological Reports 27*(1), 206.

MacDonald, A.P., Jr. (1972). Internal-external locus of control change techniques. *Rehabilitation Literature 33*(2), 44–47.

Marston, M.V. (1970). Compliance with medical regimens: A review of the literature. *Nursing Research 19*(4), 312–321.

Mazzullo, J., Lasagna, L., & Griner, P. (1974). Variations in interpretations of prescriptions. *Journal of the American Medical Association 227*(8), 929–931.

McCusker, J., & Morrow, J. (1979). The relationship of health locus of control to preventive health behaviors and health behaviors. *Patient Counselling and Health Education 1*(4), 146–150.

Meyer, D., Leventhal, H., & Gutmann, M. *Symptoms in hypertension: How patients evaluate and treat them*. Unpublished manuscript.

Meyers, A., Dolan, T.F., Jr., & Mueller, D. (1975). Compliance and self-medication in cystic fibrosis. *American Journal of Diseases of Children 129*(9), 1011–1013.

Miller, P., Johnson, Garrett, Wickoff, & McMahon. (1982). Health beliefs of and adherence to the medical regimen by patients with ischemic heart disease. *Heart and Lung 11*(4), 332–339.

Mootz, M. (1982). Attitudes toward health in social networks: Their influence on physician utilization. *Patient Counselling and Health Education 4*(1), 44–49.

Morris, L.A., & Kanouse, D.E. (1979). Drug taking for physical symptoms. In I.H. Frieze, D. Bar-Tal, & S. Carroll (Eds.), *New approaches to social problems*. San Francisco: Jossey-Bass Pubs.

Nelson, E., Stason, W., Neutra, R., & Solomon, H. (1980). Identification of noncompliant hypertensive patients. *Preventive Medicine 9*(4), 504–517.

Ozuna, J. (1981). Compliance with therapeutic regimens: Issues, answers and research questions. *Journal of Neurosurgical Nursing 13*(1), 1–6.

Phares, E.J. (1976). *Locus of control in personality*. Morristown, NJ: General Learning Press.

Procci, W.R. (1978). Dietary abuse in maintenance hemodialysis patients. *Psychosomatics 19*(1), 16–24.

Redman, B.K. (1978). Curriculum in patient education. *American Journal of Nursing 78*(8), 1363–1366.

Rokeach, M. (1973). *The nature of human values*. New York: The Free Press.

Rokeach, M. (1980). *Beliefs, attitudes and values*. San Francisco: Jossey-Bass Pubs.

Rotter, J. (1966). Generalized expectancies for internal versus external control of reinforcement [entire issue]. *Psychological Monographs: General and Applied 80* (609).

Rudy, E.B. (1980). Patients' and spouses' causal explanations of myocardial infarction. *Nursing Research 29*(6), 352–356.

Sackett, D., Haynes, R., Gibson, E., Taylor, D., Roberts, R., & Johnson, A. (1978). Patient compliance with antihypertensive regimens. *Patient Counselling and Health Education 1*(1), 18–21.

Samora, J., Saunders, L., & Larson, R. (1961). Medical vocabulary knowledge among hospital patients. *Journal of Health and Human Behavior 2*(1), 83–92.

Seeman, M., & Evans, J. (1962). Alienation and learning in a hospital setting. *American Sociological Review 27*, 772–782.

Sejwacz, D., Ajzen, I., & Fishbein, M. (1980). Predicting and understanding weight loss: Intentions, behaviors, and outcomes. In I. Ajzen & M. Fishbein (Eds.), *Understanding attitudes and predicting social behavior*. Englewood Cliffs, NJ: Prentice-Hall, Inc.

Shaver, K.G. (1975). *An introduction to the attribution process*. Cambridge, MA: Winthrop.

Schillinger, F.L. (1983). Locus of control: Implications for clinical nursing practice. *Image: The Journal of Nursing Scholarship 15*(2), 58–63.

Stanitis, M.A., & Ryan, J. (1982). Noncompliance: An unacceptable diagnosis? *American Journal of Nursing 82*(6), 941–942.

Starfield, B., Wray, C., Hess, K., Gross, R., Birk, P., & D'Lugoff, B. (1981). The influence of patient-practitioner agreement on outcome of care. *American Journal of Public Health 71*(2), 127–130.

Stillman, M.J. (1977). Women's health beliefs about breast cancer and breast self examination. *Nursing Research 26*(2), 121–127.

Suchman, E. (1970). Health attitudes and behavior. *Archives of Environmental Health 20*(1), 105–110.

Tirrell, B., & Hart, L. (1980). The relationships of health beliefs and knowledge to exercise compliance in patients after coronary bypass. *Heart and Lung 9*(3), 487–493.

Vertinsky, P., Yang, C., MacLeod, P., & Hardwick, D. (1976). A study of compliance factors in voluntary health behaviour. *International Journal of Health Education 19*(1), 16–28.

Wallston, K., Maides, S., & Wallston, B. (1976). Health related information seeking as a function of health related locus of control and health value. *Journal of Research in Psychology 10*(2), 215–222.

Wallston, B., Wallston, K., Kaplan, G., & Maides, S. (1976). Development and validation of the health locus of control scale. *Journal of Consulting and Clinical Psychology 44*(4), 580–585.

Watts, D. (1966). Factors related to the acceptance of modern medicine. *American Journal of Public Health 56*(8), 1205–1212.

Wooley, F.R., Kane, R.L., Hughes, C.C., & Wright, D. (1978). The effects of doctor-patient communication on satisfaction and outcome of care. *Social Science and Medicine 12*(2A), 123–128.

SUGGESTED READINGS

Aho, W. (1977). Relationship of wives' preventive health orientation to their beliefs about heart disease in husbands. *Public Health Reports 92*(1), 65–71.

Ajzen, I., & Fishbein, M. (1974). Factors influencing intentions and the intention-behavior relation. *Human Relations 27*(1), 1–15.

Andrew, J.M. (1972). Delay of surgery. *Psychosomatic Medicine 34*(4), 345–354.

Arakelian, M. (1980). An assessment and nursing application of the concept of locus of control. *Advances in Nursing Science 3*(1), 25–42.

Barofsky, I. (1978). Compliance, adherence and the therapeutic alliance: Steps in the development of self care. *Social Science and Medicine 12*(5A), 369–376.

Battle, E.H., Halliburton, A., & Wallston, K.A. (1982). Self-medication among psychiatric patients and adherence after discharge. *Journal of Psychosocial Nursing and Mental Health Services 20*(5), 21–28.

Becker, M., Haefner, D., Kasl, S., Kirscht, J., Maiman, L., & Rosenstock, I. (1977). Selected psychological models and correlates of individual health related behaviors [supplement]. *Medical Care 15*(15), 27–46.

Becker, M., Kaback, M., Rosenstock, I., & Ruth, M. (1975). Some influences on public participation in a genetic screening program. *Journal of Community Health 1*(1), 3–14.

Becker, M., Maiman, L., Kirscht, J., Haefner, D., & Drachman, R. (1977). The health belief model and prediction of dietary compliance: A field experiment. *Journal of Health and Social Behavior 18*(4), 348–366.

Becker, M., Radius, S., Rosenstock, I., Drachman, R., Schuberth, K., & Teets, K. (1978). Compliance with a medical regimen for asthma: A test of the health belief model. *Public Health Reports 93*(3), 268–277.

Berkanovic, E., & Telesky, C. (1982). Social networks, beliefs and the decision to seek medical care: An analysis of congruent and incongruent patterns. *Medical Care 20*(10), 1018–1026.

Bowler, M., Morisky, D., & Deeds, S. (1980). Needs assessment strategies in working with compliance issues and blood pressure control. *Patient Counselling and Health Education 2*(1), 22–27.

Cohen, S. (1981). Patient education: A review of the literature. *Journal of Advanced Nursing 6*, 11–18.

Cowie, B. (1976). The cardiac patient's perception of his heart attack. *Social Science and Medicine 10*, 87–96.

Cummings, K.M., Becker, M.H., Kirscht, J., & Levin, N. (1982). Psychosocial factors affecting adherence to medical regimens in a group of hemodialysis patients. *Medical Care 20*(6), 567–580.

Cummings, K.M., Jette, A.M., & Rosenstock, I.M. (1978). Construct validation of the health belief model. *Health Education Monographs 6*(4), 394–405.

Davis, M., & Eichhorn, R. (1963). Compliance with medical regimens: A panel study. *Journal of Health and Human Behavior 4*(4), 240–249.

de Haes, W.F. (1982). Patient education: A component of health education. *Patient Counselling and Health Education 4*(2), 95–102.

Dielman, T.E. (1982). Parental and child health beliefs and behavior. *Health Education Quarterly 9*(2 & 3), 60–77, 156–173.

Elder, R.G. (1973). Social class and lay explanations of the etiology of arthritis. *Journal of Health and Human Behavior 14*(1), 28–38.

Fishbein, M. (1980). A theory of reasoned action: Some applications and implications. In M. Howe & M. Page (Eds.), *The 1979 Nebraska symposium on motivation 27*, 65–116.

Frieze, I.H., & Bar-Tal, D. (1979). Attribution theory: Past and present. In I.H. Frieze, D. Bar-Tal, & S. Carroll (Eds.), *New approaches to social problems*. San Francisco: Jossey-Bass Pubs.

Glanz, K., Kirscht, J., & Rosenstock, I. (1981). Initial knowledge and attitudes as predictors of intervention effects: The individual management plan. *Patient Counselling and Health Education 3*(1), 30–41.

Gochman, D. (1972). The organizing role of motivation in health beliefs and intentions. *Journal of Health and Social Behavior 13*(3), 285–293.

Gottlieb, B. (Ed.). (1983). *Social networks and social support*. Beverly Hills: Sage Publications.

Green, L.W. (1970). Should health education abandon attitude change strategies? Perspectives from recent research. *Health Education Monographs 30*, 25–48.

Green, L.W., Kreuter, M., Deeds, S., & Partridge, K. (1980). *Health education planning: A diagnostic approach*. Palo Alto, CA: Mayfield Publishing.

Green, L.W., Levine, D., & Deeds, S. (1975). Clinical trials of health education for hypertensive outpatients: Design and baseline data. *Preventive Medicine 4*(4), 417–425.

Harris, D.M., & Guten, S. (1979). Health protective behavior: An exploratory study. *Journal of Health and Social Behavior 20*(1), 17–29.

Harvey, J.H., Ickes, W., & Kidd, R.F. (Eds.). (1976, 1978, 1981). *New directions in attribution research* (vols. 1, 2, & 3). Hillsdale, NJ: Lawrence Erlbaum Associates.

Hayes-Bautista, D. (1976). Modifying the treatment: Patient compliance, patient control and medical care. *Social Science and Medicine 10*(5), 233–238.

Haynes, J., & Mathews, B. (1974). Human values: Implications for health education practice. *International Journal of Health Education 17*(4), 266–273.

Haynes, R.B., Taylor, D.W., & Sackett, D. (Eds.). (1979). *Compliance in health care*. Baltimore: Johns Hopkins University Press.

Hefferin, E.A. (1977). Patient health education: Goal or element in modern health care. *Health Values 1*(2), 66–72.

Horan, M.L. (1982). Parental reaction to the birth of an infant with a defect: An attributional approach. *Advances in Nursing Science 5*(1), 57–68.

Ickes, W., & Layden, M.A. (1978). Attributional styles. In W. Ickes & R.F. Kidds (Eds.), *New directions in attribution research*. Hillsdale, NJ: Lawrence Erlbaum Associates.

Inui, T., Carter, W., & Pecoraro, R. (1981). Screening for noncompliance among patients with hypertension: Is self-report the best available measure? *Medical Care 19*(10), 1061–1064.

Janis, I., & Rodin, J. (1980). Attribution, control and decision making: Social psychology and health care. In G. Stone, F. Cohen, & N. Adler (Eds.), *Health psychology*. San Francisco: Jossey-Bass Pubs.

Jenny, J. (1978). A strategy for patient teaching. *Journal of Advanced Nursing 3*(4), 341–348.

Jones, E., Kanouse, D., Kelley, H., Nisbett, R., Valins, S., & Weiner, B. (1971). *Attribution: Perceiving the causes of behavior*. Morristown, NJ: General Learning Press.

Kasl, S.V. (1974). The health belief model and behavior related to chronic illness. In M. Becker (Ed.), *The health belief model and personal health behavior*. Thorofare, NJ: Charles B. Slack.

Kasl, S.V., & Cobb, S. (1966). Health behavior, illness behavior and sick role behavior: Parts I & II. *Archives of Environmental Health 12*(4), 531–541.

Kelley, H.H. (1972). Causal schemata and the attribution process. In E. Jones, D. Kanouse, H. Kelley, R. Nisbett, S. Valins, & B. Weiner (Eds.), *Attribution: Perceiving the causes of behavior*. Morristown, NJ: General Learning Press.

Kelley, H.H., & Michela, J.L. (1980). Attribution and research. *Annual Review of Psychology 31*, 457–501.

King, J. (1982). The impact of patients' perceptions of high blood pressure on attendance at screening: An extension of the health belief model. *Social Science and Medicine 16*, 1079–1091.

Kirscht, J.P. (1974). The health belief model and illness behavior. In M. Becker (Ed.), *The health belief model and personal health behavior*. Thorofare, NJ: Charles B. Slack.

Kirscht, J.P., Haefner, D., Kegeles, S., & Rosenstock, I. (1966). A national study of health beliefs. *Journal of Health and Human Behavior 7*(4), 248–254.

Knox, R. (1984, January 23). Lowering cholesterol helps heart *The Boston Globe*, p. 41.

Kopel, S., & Arkowitz, H. (1975). The role of attribution and self-perception in behavior change. *Genetic Psychology Monographs 92*, 175–212.

Leavitt, F. (1979). The health belief model and utilization of ambulatory care services. *Social Science and Medicine 13A*(1), 105–112.

Leventhal, H. (1970). Findings and theory in the study of fear communications. In L. Berkowitz (Ed.), *Advances in experimental social psychology* (vol. 5). New York: Academic Press.

Leventhal, H., Meyer, D., & Nerenz, D. (1980). The commonsense representation of illness danger. In S. Rachman (Ed.), *Contributions to medical psychology* (vol. 2). Oxford: Pergamon Press.

Leventhal, H., Safer, M., & Panagis, D. (1983). The impact of communications on the self-regulation of health beliefs, decisions and behavior. *Health Education Quarterly 10*(1), 3–30.

Loustau, A. (1979). Using the health belief model to predict patient compliance. *Health Values 3*, 242–245.

Lowery, B.J. (1981). Misconceptions and limitations of locus of control and the I-E scale. *Nursing Research 30*(5), 294–298.

Lowery, B.J., & DuCette, J. (1976). Disease related learning and disease control in diabetes as a function of locus of control. *Nursing Research 25*(5), 358–362.

Lowery, B.J., Jackson, B.S., & Murphy, B.B. (1983). An exploratory investigation of the causal thinking of arthritics. *Nursing Research 32*(3), 157–162.

Mabry, J.H. (1964). Lay concepts of etiology. *Journal of Chronic Diseases 17*, 371–386.

MacDonald, A.P., Jr. (1971). Perception of disability by the disabled. *Journal of Consulting and Clinical Psychology 36*(3), 338–343.

Maiman, L.A., & Becker, M. (1974). The health belief model: Origins and correlates in psychological theory. In M. Becker (Ed.), *The health belief model and personal health behavior*. Thorofare, NJ: Charles B. Slack.

Marston, M.V. (1978). The use of knowledge. In M. Hardy & M. Conway (Eds.), *Role theory: Perspectives for health professionals*. New York: Appleton-Century-Crofts.

Mechanic, D. (1962). The concept of illness behavior. *Journal of Chronic Diseases 15*, 189.

Mechanic, D. (1966). Response factors in illness: The study of illness behavior. *Social Psychiatry 1*, 11–20.

Mechanic, D. (1972). Social psychological factors affecting the presentation of bodily complaints. *New England Journal of Medicine 286*(21), 1132–1139.

Mikhail, B. (1981). The health belief model: A review and critical evaluation of the model, research and practice. *Advances in Nursing Science 4*(1), 65–80.

Murray, R., & Zentner, J. (1976). Guidelines for more effective health teaching. *Nursing 76 6*(2), 44–53.

Naisbitt, J. (1982). *Megatrends: Ten new directions transforming our lives*. New York: Warner Books.

Phares, E.J., Ritchie, D.E., & Davis, W.L. (1968). I-E control and reaction to threat. *Journal of Personality and Social Psychology 10*(4), 402–405.

Redman, B.K. (1976). *The process of patient teaching in nursing*. St. Louis: C.V. Mosby Co.

Rodin, J. (1978). Somatophysics and attribution. *Perspectives of Psychology Bulletin 4*(4), 531–540.

Rosenstock, I. (1966). Why people use health services. *Milbank Memorial Fund Quarterly 44*(3, part 2), 94–124.

Rosenstock, I. (1974). The health belief model and preventive health behavior. In M. Becker (Ed.), *The health belief model and personal health behavior*. Thorofare, NJ: Charles B. Slack.

Rosenstock, I. (1974). Historical origins of the health belief model. In M. Becker (Ed.), *The health belief model and personal health behavior*. Thorofare, NJ: Charles B. Slack.

Rosenstock, I., & Kirscht, J. (1980). Why people seek health care. In G. Stone, F. Cohen, & N. Adler (Eds.), *Health psychology*. San Francisco: Jossey-Bass Pubs.

Rotter, J., Chance, J., & Phares, E. (1972). *Applications of a social learning theory of personality*. New York: Holt, Rinehart & Winston, Inc.

Scherwitz, L., & Leventhal, H. (1978). Strategies for increasing patient compliance. *Health Values 2*(6), 301–306.

Simonds, S. (1983). Individual health counselling and education: Emerging directions from current theory, research and practice. *Patient Counselling and Health Education 4*(4), 175–181.

Smith, B., & Carson, H. (1981). The relationship of health locus of control to patients with end stage renal disease. *Patient Counselling and Health Education 3*(2), 63–66.

Storms, M., & Nisbett, R. (1970). Insomnia and the attribution process. *Journal of Personality and Social Psychology 16*(2), 319–328.

Suchman, E. (1965*a*). Social patterns of illness and medical care. *Journal of Health and Human Behavior 6*(1), 2–16.

Suchman, E. (1965*b*). Stages of illness and medical care. *Journal of Health and Human Behavior 6*(3), 114–128.

Suls, J., & Sanders, J. (Eds.). (1982). *Social psychology of health and illness*. Hillsdale, NJ: Lawrence Erlbaum Associates.

Tagliacozzo, D.M., & Ima, K. (1970). Knowledge of illness as a predictor of patient behavior. *Journal of Chronic Diseases 22*(11), 765–775.

Tagliacozzo, D.M., Luskin, D.B., Lashof, J.C., & Ima, K. (1974). Nurse intervention and patient behavior: An experimental study. *American Journal of Public Health 64*(6), 596–603.

Villeneuve, M.E. (1982). The patient compliance puzzle. *Nursing Management 13*(5), 54–56.

Wallston, B., & Wallston, K. (1978). Locus of control and health: A review of literature. *Health Education Monographs 6*, 107–117.

Wallston, K., Wallston, B., & DeVellis, R. (1978). Development of the multidimensional health locus of control scales. *Health Education Monographs 6*(2), 160–170.

Ware, J., Jr. (1976). Scales for measuring general health perceptions. *Health Services Research 11*(4), 396–415.

Wartman, S.A., Morlock, L.L., Malitz, F.E., & Palm, E.A. (1983). Patient understanding and satisfaction as predictors of compliance. *Medical Care 21*(9), 886–891.

Weiner, B. (Ed.). (1974). *Cognitive views of human motivation*. New York: Academic Press.

Wineman, N.M. (1980). Obesity: Locus of control, body image, weight loss and age-at-onset. *Nursing Research 29*(4), 231–237.

Zola, I.K. (1966). Culture and symptoms: An analysis of patients' presenting complaints. *American Sociological Review 31*(5), 615–680.

Zola, I.K. (1972). Studying the decision to see a doctor. In Z.J. Lipowski (Ed.), *Advances in psychosomatic medicine*. New York: S. Karger.

Chapter 4

Interpersonal Techniques and Teaching Strategies

Karyl M. Woldum, RN, BSN, MSN

It is important that every nurse enter a teaching situation intent on building and evolving a working relationship with the patient. A relationship implies two people working together. As a teaching and learning relationship develops, the nurse and patient negotiate to outline mutual learning goals and eventually agree on objectives, type of instruction, educational tools, and a reasonable time table for learning. In other words the nurse and the patient develop a contract.

This process—establishing a relationship, negotiating for mutual goals, and finally agreeing on a learning contract—is part of every teaching situation. At times the process may be more structured or formal than others, but if the process of building a relationship is not completed, education is difficult, if not impossible, for the nurse and the patient may be working against each other rather than with each other.

ESTABLISHMENT OF A RELATIONSHIP

In order to ensure success in a teacher and learner interaction, the dynamics of a relationship must be understood and the interaction considered in terms of a productive relationship. The type of communication between provider and patient contributes heavily to the feeling of satisfaction that a patient has about health care (Pool, 1980). Steckel (1982) states that the quality of interaction significantly contributes to the outcome of health care, patient knowledge, and satisfaction of medical care. Lum et al. (1978) report that the more we involve patients in their care, the more they feel the need to have things explained to them. This finding suggests that the type of relationship between a patient and nurse may trigger greater interest in participating in the treatment program.

"A relationship is a goal directed interaction between two people that is mutually determined and accepted" (Byrne & Thompson, 1978, p. 121). These

Karyl M. Woldum is Associate Chairman in the Department of Nursing at the New England Medical Center Hospitals, Boston.

authors identify and describe the three stages of every relationship: (1) the orientation stage, (2) the utilization stage, and (3) the resolution stage. These stages apply not only to the total relationship but also to every interaction within the relationship. For instance, the nurse may establish a relationship with a patient to teach care for a gastrostomy. This may require 10 teaching sessions or interactions. During each of these interactions the nurse will go through the three stages of orientation, utilization, and resolution. As both parties get to know each other, they may go through some stages so fast that they appear to be almost simultaneous (Byrne & Thompson, 1978).

Orientation Stage

Byrne & Thompson (1978) point out that the first stage, or orientation, is characterized by a testing period. The patient is deciding whether the nurse is a reliable, helping person, and the nurse may be determining the patient's ability and willingness to learn. The nurse and the patient are assessing each other. It is the period in which questions are asked and explanations and reasons are given. Both parties explore the needs and concerns of each other. They might observe: "She is funny"; "He is smart"; "He knows what he is talking about"; or "She's scared." How much information is shared may be related to how quickly a feeling of trust and security is established. As the patient's feelings of safety are developed, willingness to discuss past experiences, concerns, and problems is increased.

During this phase the goals or reasons for the relationship or interaction are established. The patient's health and learning needs perceived by the nurse are discussed. The patient identifies priorities and concerns. The two parties then negotiate mutually acceptable long- and short-term goals. In a personal relationship the short-term goal of one interaction may be to buy clothes or to eat lunch. The long-term goal is to provide ongoing support. In a nurse-patient relationship the long-term goal, or objective of the relationship, might be to take medications wisely and correctly. The short-term goal, or objective of one 5-minute interaction, might be to learn the purpose and action of the drug. The more specifically the goals are outlined, the easier it will be to measure the effectiveness of the interaction or relationship as a whole.

During the orientation stage, the benefits, duration, and conditions of the relationship are also identified (Byrne & Thompson, 1978). Every relationship has benefits for both parties that must be clearly acknowledged. Who will benefit? How will the rewards be received? The benefit to the patient may be improved health, ability to return to work, or a better self-image. The nurse may have the satisfaction of doing a job well, gain prestige from peers, or gain new knowledge about a patient care problem. It is also important that the participants of a relationship have a tentative and realistic expectation of their time involvement. They should have some understanding about the length of time that needs to be committed to achieve the goals of the relationship and each individual interaction. For example, a friendship may not have a time limitation, but during one interaction you may announce that you have 4 hours for shopping. In a business interaction, time is designated in terms of 1 hour for a meeting or 2 months to complete a project. With our patients we may have 1 week to complete our goals, or an individual teaching session may be scheduled for 5 minutes, 20 minutes, or 1 hour. The participants in a relationship need to understand what, if any, conditions or constraints are attached to the relationship. In other words, the ground rules must be established. The conditions or actions that would place the relationship in jeopardy are identified. In a teaching relationship the conditions may be that the teacher keeps the appointment to teach and that the patient tries to learn.

Included in the orientation stage, usually in the beginning of a short interaction, is a repetition or reclarification of material previously discussed. This allows both parties to reestablish or renegotiate goals that may have changed since the last interaction. The patient may be unclear about information discussed at the last interaction, or a family member may have asked why a particular treatment was necessary.

Utilization Stage

After one goes through the orientation stage, the relationship moves to the utilization stage. During this stage the nurse and the patient are working together to achieve the agreed objectives. Each interaction has short-term objectives that contribute to the achievement of the overall objectives. During this stage the nurse is not doing to the patient or doing for but doing with the patient. The more "doing with" that takes place in a teaching relationship, the better prepared the patient will be to take control once the relationship has been terminated. For instance, the patient and nurse agree to work together so that the patient is comfortably changing the dressing every day before discharge.

Resolution Stage

The final stage of the relationship described by Byrne & Thompson (1978) is the resolution stage. After a joint evaluation of the relationship, it should be terminated by mutual agreement. The evaluation includes a discussion of the objectives and how they were achieved, an identification of the strengths of the patient, and a discussion of the weak areas that may require continuing effort. Finally resources are identified that may be available to the patient after an interaction or relationship has ended. The resources may be material to be read or reviewed, or if the patient is discharged from the hospital and the relationship is permanently terminated, the outpatient nurse, visiting nurse association, or family member may be designated as a resource.

NEGOTIATION

A satisfactory relationship is built on mutual goals that provide the framework for a formal contract. What happens if the patient's goals are different from yours? How do you arrive at a mutually acceptable goal? You negotiate.

Negotiation is a means of getting what you want from others. It is important, however, that you negotiate not just for what you want but for the best agreement for both the patient and the nurse. Patients must not feel that they have been manipulated into agreeing to a goal that they aren't committed to achieving. Hughes (1980, p. 23) states that "any situation in which the learner is not participating in the identification of his learning needs and in the learning itself is destructive." If the situation is not desirable for both parties concerned, then any manipulative behavior will be destructive. Fisher and Ury (1981) have identified four basic elements that will help ensure a good negotiation: (1) people, (2) interests, (3) options, and (4) criteria.

The people element seems obvious, but too often we forget that in order to understand the action of a person, we must understand the individual. Nurses must be careful not to prejudge or assume the reasons for a patient's actions. For instance, the nurse has just told a patient that medication must be taken on a daily basis and a series of breathing exercises must be performed to treat the problem of chronic obstructive pulmonary disease. The patient wants nothing to do with this treatment regimen. Is the nurse at an impasse? Perhaps not. The nurse must start by exploring what taking medication means to the patient. Are the breathing exercises the problem? Has the medication been taken in the past? What were the consequences of that last experience? Does the patient know anyone who has chronic obstructive pulmonary disease? How do these people treat their problems? Through the discussion of these issues the nurse may be able to see the patient's point of view and understand the reason for resistance.

The second element in negotiation is interest. Often nurses enter into a negotiation with an established position. The patient states that it is impossible to take pills every day and won't do it. The nurse takes another position and counters that the medication must be taken daily or serious breathing problems will result. Instead of focusing on positions, both the patient and the nurse must find a common interest. The nurse wants the patient to stay healthy. So does the patient. How this common interest is reached remains the issue. Try to find common interests. What is your basic concern? Why doesn't the patient agree? Find something that can be agreed on. Examples should be used to show the patient why you are concerned. For instance, tell the patient that chest pain may become more severe, infection will spread, etc., without treatment. The patient's concern for security, economic well-being, a sense of belonging, recognition, or control over life style should be explored. Try to focus on the issue, not your personal preferences. For instance, you have noticed that the patient becomes short of breath after climbing one flight of stairs. The patient has grandchildren who live on the third floor. If the symptoms are relieved, the patient will be able to climb the stairs to visit them. In this case both the patient and the nurse want to relieve the patient's symptoms so that a normal routine can be maintained.

Before negotiations are begun, options should be identified. Are there other ways acceptable to both parties that will achieve the same objectives? The nurse should consider all alternatives, for there usually is more than one answer. Brainstorming, without regard for the perfect solution, is a good way to elicit options acceptable to both of you. If the patient indicates that an alternative might be acceptable, try to find a way to make the decision easier.

For example, the patient with chronic obstructive pulmonary disease might have several options. Different mechanisms might have a similar action. The patient may participate in various discussions such as how to do breathing exercises, how many to learn, when to do them.

Objective criteria on which the results of negotiation might be based are the final element. Standards that are considered fair by both parties should be identified. Possibly a standard based on the premise that the patient wants to self-help and one that will decrease symptoms would be acceptable to the patient and the nurse. Once the nurse and patient have identified the standards on which the negotiations are based, they should not yield to pressure to change these standards. For instance, the patient offers to do breathing exercises, but only once a week. To agree to this treatment modality knowing that it will not accomplish the standard of decreasing symptoms would not be appropriate.

Alternative to Negotiated Agreement

What happens if the nurse has used all these elements of people, interest, options, and criteria in a negotiation, and it still didn't work out—they couldn't come to an agreement?

Fisher and Ury (1981) suggest that you use your "best alternative to a negotiated agreement" (p. 104). This alternative should be identified before negotiations begin.

If the patient doesn't want to participate in the treatment plan, the best alternative may be family, friends, visiting nurse association, a community health center, or even extended care. The better your best alternative, the greater the nurse's power and patience with the patient during negotiations. If the nurse can easily walk away from a negotiation, the better the chances to affect its outcome objectively.

What happens if the patient stands firm and doesn't agree to work on an important learning goal? The nurse negotiates an interest and the patient sticks to a position. Patients who won't negotiate may use three maneuvers: (1) insist on their ideas, (2) attack the nurse's ideas, and (3) attack the nurse.

The nurse should neither accept nor reject the patient's position but instead try to understand the reasons behind it. Discuss what might happen if you went along with the patient's position. Don't defend your ideas, ask what is wrong with them. Then work with the patient to develop a plan that is acceptable to both of you.

FORMULATION OF A CONTRACT

Contracting is a patient-teaching technique that is based on the components of a good relationship and is formulated through negotiation.

Simply stated, a contract is a mutual agreement between two people. It may be written or verbal. Some patients and nurses initially perceive a verbal contract to be less formal and therefore less threatening than a written one. The hazard in verbal contracts may be the same as their perceived benefits, for verbal contracts can be too informal, causing both parties to lose track of their goals and responsibilities. A written contract clearly identifies goals, ensuring mutual understanding and providing a structured means to evaluate learning progress. Written contracts are not permanently binding. The nurse or the patient should feel free to renegotiate a contract if the goals seem unrealistic or the circumstances under which the contract was formulated change.

Benefits of Contracts

A contract ensures patients' participation in their own health care. The more involved in planning goals and implementing treatment modalities, the better prepared patients will be for discharge and for self-care activities at home. The patient who is knowledgeable about self-care activities and is an active participant in establishing treatment goals is more likely to follow through with the treatment plan after leaving the hospital or between outpatient visits. Thus, contracting is an effective tool in improving compliance with a medical regime or in improving health habits (Steckel, 1980).

A written contract establishes a legitimate relationship between the patient and the nurse. It is a mechanism through which a nurse and a patient can clarify expectations of one another and put away preconceived ideas. While negotiating a contract, nurses are given an opportunity to discuss their roles in providing health care and the patient can establish priorities and clarify misunderstandings.

CONTINGENCY CONTRACTING

A contingency contract is an agreement between two people that stipulates a reward or reinforcer on accomplishment of a goal (Steckel, 1982). This kind of contract is based on the premise that the patient and the nurse are equal partners and that the responsibilities of each individual are equally divided. A written contract has several elements:

- needs assessment
- goals and objectives
- responsibilities
- time schedule
- reinforcers
- evaluation

Needs Assessment

As in other teaching and learning situations, the nurse approaches contracting by evaluating the patient's readiness to learn, personal priorities, past experiences, support systems, and ability to learn. The nurse uses this assessment to determine learning priorities and to establish what must be addressed or resolved before implementing the contract. For instance, the patient and the nurse may agree to a visit from a family member or assurance from the physician about the prognosis of the problem before beginning work on the contract.

The patient's strengths and weaknesses should also be identified and considered when formulating the contract. For instance, the patient may be very adept at manual tasks but have trouble remembering new things. In the past a list has been helpful to the patient as new tasks were conquered. The two of you have identified a need to learn how to change a dressing. Based on the assessment, a contract is drawn in which the nurse agrees to provide a diagram and a step-by-step written outline describing how to change a dressing.

The nurse and the patient gain information during the assessment that will help them formulate a contract based on realistic expectations of both parties. The nurse must keep one factor in mind: although information is given to the patient to help establish goals, the decision about what is to be learned, how it is to be taught, and when learning is to take place is ultimately made by the patient.

Goals and Objectives

After the needs assessment is completed, the patient and the nurse must agree on the goals of a contract. Even if the patient has multiple learning needs, it is wise to start small and focus initially on one goal. Once both of you have had success in achieving the first learning need, you will be more willing to try contracting again. The teaching plans in this book may be useful tools in helping patients to think about goals.

The goals of the written contract should be outlined in terms of long-term objectives and shorter-term objectives, whose accomplishment leads to the completion of the long-term goal much like the informal goals of any relationship. The goals should be stated in behavioral terms describing what a patient will be doing to demonstrate accomplishment of the goal. In other words, the goal should be both measurable and observable. For instance, instead of writing that "the patient understands the signs of infection," the goal should be stated as "the patient describes three signs and symptoms of infection from memory."

The patient and the nurse have agreed that an appropriate long-term goal is to change the dressing on a vascular ulcer at home. To help the patient achieve this goal, short-term goals are outlined; their accomplishment is a series of stepping stones to the achievement of the long-term goal. Examples include the following:

- The patient describes the purpose of the dressing.
- The patient identifies the supplies needed to change the dressing.
- The patient demonstrates clean technique.
- The patient describes how to change the dressing and demonstrates the dressing change correctly.
- The patient changes the dressing correctly three times.

It is useless to set goals that are not realistically achievable because they won't be completed in the time available. Assure both yourself and your patient success by establishing a meaningful, realistic contract.

Responsibilities

In addition to identifying the goals of the contract, the responsibilities of both the patient and the nurse in achieving the goals must be stipulated. It is important that these activities be specific and directed to the accomplishment of each short-term goal. If a choice of several activities is an option, all these alternatives should be identified (Exhibit 4–1).

Time Schedule

After the goals of the contract are identified and the responsibilities of each party are outlined, a specific time schedule should be developed for completion of the long- and short-term goals. Discuss when work can begin. Perhaps some learning

Exhibit 4–1 Sample Goal and Responsibilities

Goal	Patient Responsibilities	Nurse Responsibilities
The patient describes the purpose of the dressing.	1. Reads handout.	1. Discusses the purpose as the dressing is changed.
	2. Is available after dinner for dressing change.	2. Leaves handout for the patient to read.
		3. Is available for clarification for 10 minutes after dinner.

can take place now; other goals may be postponed for a day or a week. Determine what can realistically be accomplished in the time open to you. Then be specific; consider the number of teaching sessions and the duration of each session.

For instance, if the nurse has 3 days to teach a patient to change the dressing, the number and length of the sessions should be identified and a schedule outlined considering the time available.

Reinforcers

Once the contract has been agreed upon, reinforcers or rewards for accomplishing identified goals should be stipulated. Steckel (1982) describes a reinforcer as any consequence that strengthens behavior. Many nurses are uncomfortable about giving rewards to patients in return for something that they should be doing anyway. In fact when asked to designate a reward, some patients may respond that achieving the goal is its own reward.

The patient, however, should try very hard to think of a reward because the use of reinforcers is based on the educational principle that behaviors that are reinforced are more likely to be sustained or increased. Behaviors are greatly influenced by their rewards.

A reward can be something desired and given as a consequence of behavior. However, if it does not increase the probability of sustaining the behavior, it is not a reinforcer (Steckel, 1982). Reinforcers may not always remain the same. Often the reinforcer originally chosen may no longer be effective in maintaining or increasing a behavior, so a new reinforcer must be chosen.

Types of Reinforcers

How does the nurse help the patient choose reinforcers? First, a specific reinforcer should be stipulated for each goal. A reinforcer should be something that a patient likes or wants, for instance, an extra snack, back rubs, a visit, a new watch, tickets to a play, or extra time spent with the nurse. It is sometimes helpful to ask patients to recall situations when they might have used rewards in order to explain their usefulness in a contract. People frequently promise themselves rewards when they want to change an important behavior. For instance, a woman may promise herself a new dress for losing 10 pounds or a special vacation for successfully giving up smoking. Parents have also found rewards helpful in changing the behavior of children. Dessert is promised if the dinner meal is eaten, or a new watch is given to the child if thumb sucking is conquered.

Rewards may also be cumulative. For example, points might be earned toward a larger reward. A graph showing progress might also be used. Children are often given stars of different colors, and the winner may then earn a set of colored pencils or a box of crayons.

Evaluation

Written contracts are easy to evaluate as learning progresses because expected behaviors and responsibilities are clearly delineated. If either the nurse or the patient does not meet responsibilities, the problems can be identified early.

If an individual is unable to fulfill the agreed responsibilities, an alternative plan is sometimes worthwhile. For instance, if a patient becomes more acutely ill or overwhelmed, the time scheduled might be altered or the contract might be modified to include the family. If the nurse finds the responsibilities impossible to complete, a peer might be asked to assist in meeting the responsibilities.

When To Use Contracts

Contracting is a useful tool with a wide variety of patients. Patients with chronic diseases such as renal failure, hypertension, or chronic obstructive pulmonary disease may benefit from a contract. Many times the behavior changes with which they must deal are overwhelming. Through the process of contracting, patients gain a feeling of success from accomplishing goals, and since contracts are between two parties, they may not feel as alone in dealing with their problems.

Contracts are also useful in helping patients change health habits such as cessation of smoking, weight reduction, or change in dietary habits.

A contract can take many forms. A more specific contract is depicted in Exhibit 4–2. A more general contract using a patient teaching plan is depicted in Exhibit 4–3. Often patients can't meet all the objectives on one teaching plan, but they might want to select one or two on which they would like to concentrate more fully. Using the objectives selected, the nurse and the patient can delineate responsibilities, time schedule, and rewards. Despite the many possible forms, however, they all should delineate the responsibility of the patient and the nurse and include a signature of both parties. Finally each participant in the contract should receive a copy for easy reference.

Exhibit 4–2 Example of a Patient Contract

Mrs. Smith, 56-year-old female: history of varicose veins

Short-term goal: During hospitalization Mrs. Smith will perform her own vascular foot care twice daily.

Long-term goal: Mrs. Smith will do vascular foot care twice daily as part of daily activity of care.

	Nursing Responsibilities	*Patient Responsibilities*
Day 1		
8 AM	RN demonstrates foot care, organizes supplies, gives verbal explanation.	Mrs. Smith meets with RN at bedside and observes foot care.
8 PM	RN does foot care.	Mrs. Smith gives verbal description of foot care as RN does the care.
Day 2		
8 AM	RN organizes supplies, assists Mrs. Smith in doing foot care.	Mrs. Smith gives verbal explanation of foot care, assists RN do the foot care.
8 PM	RN supervises Mrs. Smith doing foot care.	Mrs. Smith does foot care.
Day 3		
8 AM	RN supervises Mrs. Smith doing foot care.	Mrs. Smith does foot care alone.
8 PM	RN checks Mrs. Smith's care.	Mrs. Smith does foot care alone.
Day 4		
8 AM	RN meets with Mrs. Smith to review contract and adjust care for home schedule.	Mrs. Smith meets with RN to review contract and adjust care for home schedule.

RN signature ____________________ Patient signature ____________________

Date ____________________ Date ____________________

Adapted by Joan Kraus.

TEACHING STRATEGIES

After the nurse and patient have developed a relationship and negotiated a contract based on mutual goals, appropriate teaching strategies must be identified to accomplish the goal. The strategies a nurse chooses to use will depend on the characteristics of the learner, the skill and preference of the nurse, the time and resources available, and the learning needs.

The goal of teaching may be to allay anxiety, build skills, or create new attitudes. A nurse teaching healthy patients about prevention and early detection of disease through instruction about the early warning signs of cancer or a self-breast exam exemplifies this type of teaching. The focus of teaching during an acute

Exhibit 4–3 Contract Using a Teaching Plan

Learning Need

To recognize and treat angina knowledgeably at home.

Nurse's Responsibilities

I, ______________________, R.N., will spend at least 10 minutes each day for the next four days reviewing the Angina Teaching Plan with Mrs. Smith.

Patient's Responsibilities

I will meet the objectives of the Angina Teaching Plan. In return for achieving my goal, I will receive a book of my choice.

____

Patient's Signature

Alternatives

If additional teaching is needed, the help of another registered nurse will be obtained.

Source: Adapted from M.E. Zangari and P. Duffy, Contracting with patients in day-to-day practice, *American Journal of Nursing* 80(3), 451–454.

illness is directed at helping the patient adjust to new stresses and understand the process of diagnosis and treatment. When patients are initially admitted to the hospital, they are acquainted with their environment, hospital routines, and communication devices. To lessen anxiety and gain cooperation, they are taught about diagnostic tests and other procedures that will be performed.

As patients become well enough to assume responsibility for their own treatment plans, nurses teach to ensure that they have the knowledge and skill to care for themselves safely. By means of instruction, nurses relinquish control to patients. Patients are taught how to administer their own medication, test their urine, or change a dressing.

When choosing a teaching strategy to fit the need and characteristics of the patient, the nurse must decide if the learning deficit is cognitive (knowledge), affective (feelings or attitude), or psychomotor (manual skill) in nature. It is also wise to consider the advantages and disadvantages of several alternative strategies. This chapter describes a few strategies in detail. A chart of these and additional strategies is displayed in Exhibit 4–4.

Programmed Instruction

"Programmed instruction is a written sequential presentation of learning steps requiring the learner to answer questions about the material presented and telling him whether he is right or wrong" (Redman, 1980, p. 152). Programs are designed to allow students to learn by themselves in settings that they choose and at their own pace. It provides them with immediate reinforcement by telling the right answer.

Exhibit 4–4 Teaching Strategies

Teaching Strategy	*Advantages*	*Disadvantages*	*Type of Learning*	*Type of Patient*
Lecture	1. Efficiency 2. No limit to the number of people	1. Less interaction 2. May be boring 3. Should be accompanied by other methods	1. Imparts new knowledge 2. Increases awareness	1. Patients who need general knowledge (new mothers) 2. Large groups of patients
Self-Monitoring	1. Makes patient aware of behavior 2. Provides specific measures	1. Requires time 2. Patient must be committed to recording behavior	1. Rearranges priorities 2. Creates new attitudes 3. Increases awareness	1. Patients who must change behavior through increased awareness (weight reduction, smoking cessation)
Role Play	1. Allows exploration of alternative ways of acting 2. Learner can see how others might do it 3. Keeps learner involved	1. Requires time 2. All participants must put themselves in the situation 3. Participants must feel they can trust one another	1. Teaches ideas and attitudes 2. Diagnoses readiness 3. Achieves understanding and insight 4. Stimulates new ideas	1. Patients with chronic disease (diabetes, hypertension) 2. Patients learning new interactions (how to direct home health aide or explain problem to friend)
Case Problems	1. Applies information to real situations 2. Provides concreteness 3. Learning is problem centered	1. Effectiveness depends on teacher 2. Some significant facts may be missing	1. Applies knowledge 2. Diagnoses problems	1. Patients who must apply knowledge (patient with angina, diabetes; new mothers)

Exhibit 4–4 continued

Teaching Strategy	*Advantages*	*Disadvantages*	*Type of Learning*	*Type of Patient*
Demonstration/ Return Demonstration	1. Presents standards for performance 2. Is visual and oral 3. Allows learner to know it can be done	1. May be difficult to see 2. Limited to small group 3. Patient may be nervous	1. Builds skills 2. Changes attitudes 3. Presents standards	1. Patients who must learn new skills (tracheostomy care, colostomy care) 2. Patients who need to understand cause and effect
Contracting	1. Ensures learner involvement 2. Promotes learner's strengths 3. Assists in identifying acceptable learning strategies	1. May be threatening 2. Requires learner decision-making 3. Is time-consuming	1. Promotes understanding 2. Changes attitudes	1. Patients with chronic disease 2. Well patients who wish to change health habits
Use of Significant Other	1. Provides learner support and reinforcement by influential person 2. Learning continues at home	1. Significant other must be willing to help 2. Significant other may be negative influence 3. Significant other may foster dependence	1. Builds skills 2. Changes attitudes 3. Reinforces standards	1. Patients who are elderly or disabled 2. Patients whose compliance is in question
Past Experiences	1. Builds on previous learning experience 2. Identifies potential problems	1. Depends on ability to recall 2. Requires insight	1. Promotes understanding 2. Creates awareness	1. Patients who are anxious or overwhelmed 2. Patients who must take medication, change behavior (diet, exercise)

Group Teaching	1. Efficient and economical 2. Participants support each other 3. Participants are actively involved	1. Group may digress 2. Some cultural mores discourage open sharing of issues 3. Transportation may be problem 4. Difficult to agree on time	1. Explores meaning 2. Increases motivation 3. Creates interest and new attitudes 4. Promotes understanding	1. Families and participants with common learning needs 2. Participants with chronic disease 3. Preoperative patients 4. School-age children
Programmed Instruction	1. Active learner participation 2. Individual pacing 3. Provides immediate feedback	1. May be boring or impersonal 2. Lack of 1:1 instruction 3. Learner must be literate 4. Learner must be self-motivated	1. Imparts knowledge 2. Develops skills	1. Patients with chronic disease (dialysis patient) 2. Patients with health promotion needs (teach diet, child safety, self-breast exam)
Games Simulation	1. Involves participants in the learning 2. Nonthreatening 3. Allows patient to use knowledge previously learned	1. Some participants dislike competition 2. Some participants have difficulty abstracting ideas or following directions 3. Some participants don't like games	1. Creates new attitudes 2. Applies knowledge	1. Adults and children with acute problems (broken bones), chronic problems (asthma, heart disease), or health promotion issues (dental care)
Tests	1. Evaluates learner's knowledge 2. Raises learner's consciousness of information they are unaware of 3. Gives a feeling of accomplishment	1. May make patients anxious 2. Time-consuming	1. Applies knowledge 2. Creates awareness	1. Adults and children who must apply knowledge (diabetic patient, surgical patient with a dressing, patient with a tracheostomy)

Exhibit 4–4 continued

Teaching Strategy	*Advantages*	*Disadvantages*	*Type of Learning*	*Type of Patient*
Printed Handouts	1. Promotes consistency 2. Gives visual reinforcement	1. Must be accompanied by verbal teaching 2. Difficult to write clearly and simply	1. Building skills 2. Imparts knowledge	1. Well patients (health maintenance literature) 2. Patients who must remember detailed information (titrating medications or difficult procedures)
Drama	1. Recreates real-life situations 2. Helps patients explore feelings	1. Requires planning and rehearsing 2. May require costumes, etc. 3. Patient must pay attention	1. Creates new attitudes 2. Stimulates new ideas 3. Achieves understanding	1. Children 2. Adults with a chronic problem (hypertension, dialysis, colostomy)
Diagrams	1. Offers visual reinforcement 2. Shows proportions and relationships 3. Attracts attention 4. Offers direct application of skills	1. Must be an accurate depiction 2. May require artistic skill to produce	1. Teaches new skills 2. Achieves understanding	1. Preschoolers 2. People with limited reading or vocabulary levels
Models	1. Encourages patient participation 2. Offers direct application of skill	1. May be expensive	1. Applies knowledge and skills 2. Promotes understanding	1. School-age children 2. Adults practicing a skill (CPR, self-breast exam, bathing a child)

Play	1. Stimulates and organizes cognitive thinking 2. Helps child move toward real world	1. Child must be healthy enough to play 2. Child must be able to give attention to play	1. Increases awareness 2. Achieves understanding 3. Stimulates new ideas	1. Children who undergo diagnostic tests, surgery
Films	1. Recreates real-life situations 2. Effective for patients with limited reading skills	1. Too fast for older people 2. May be expensive 3. Takes time to set up and run	1. Changes attitudes 2. Builds skills 3. Imparts knowledge	1. Groups of patients

"Programmed instruction takes advantage of the basic human drive for success" (Espich & Williams, 1967). Each time students make the correct response, positive reinforcement is given and the drive for success is satisfied. Each time the drive for success is satisfied, the probability increases that the correct response will be given again in a similar situation.

Programs are designed using the following method (Espich & Williams, 1967):

- The stimulus or question is presented to the learner.
- The learner is helped to make the right response to the question through clues leading toward the correct response or by telling the right answer itself.
- When the learner gives the answer, it is confirmed or corrected immediately.

Espich and Williams (1967) describe five levels of learning that may be included in a program:

1. Exposure level. At the exposure level, usually no question is associated with the material. Background information that is not necessary to remember is presented.
2. Recognition level. At this level the learner is asked to recognize an answer when it is presented with others. The patient may be asked to pick symptoms of hypoglycemia when they are presented with a group of symptoms.
3. Recall level. The learner is asked to define a term using one's own words. The patient may be asked to describe the problem or diagnosis in simple terms.
4. Memory level. At this level the learner is required to use exact words. For example, the patient may be asked to "state exactly" the dosage of insulin to be taken.
5. Concept level. The concept level asks the learner to use new information to solve a problem. The patient may be asked to describe the proper response to a fever.

One of the more frequently used types of programmed instruction is the discrimination frame sequence (Exhibit 4–5). This sequence consists of three basic frames:

1. The learner is given the correct answer and is then asked to use that knowledge to discriminate among the choices given.
2. The correct answer is removed and the learner is asked to select the correct answer from the choices given.
3. The student is asked to supply the right answer without help.

Exhibit 4–5 Discrimination Frame Sequence

1. Digoxin is used to improve the strength of the heart or to control the rate of the heartbeat.

   From the list below check those items that describe what digoxin is used for.

_____	A. Control the heart rate	_____	D. Relax muscles
_____	B. Treat infection	_____	E. Decrease temperature
_____	C. Cure a headache	_____	F. Strengthen the heartbeat

   CONFIRMATION:

   The correct response is _X_ A. Control the heart rate
   _X_ F. Strengthen the heartbeat

---

2. Digoxin is used to (check the correct answers):

_____	A. Improve eyesight	_____	D. Relieve stomach distress
_____	B. Strengthen the heartbeat	_____	E. Speed the heart rate
_____	C. Control the heart rate	_____	F. Relax muscles

   CONFIRMATION:

   The correct response is _X_ B. Strengthen the heartbeat
   _X_ C. Control the heart rate

---

3. Give two reasons for the use of digoxin:

   1.

   2.

   CONFIRMATION:

   The correct response is _X_ 1. Strengthen the heartbeat
   _X_ 2. Control the rate of the heart

Programmed instruction may not be appropriate for individuals whose attention span is limited or who are not motivated to learn in isolation. Some patients find it boring and impersonal. For those patients who have visual problems, it may also be difficult. It is, however, a method that many patients enjoy, for it offers an independent learning situation with immediate feedback. The nurse should keep in mind that this method, like most methods, needs opportunity for discussion and clarification.

Games

We are always looking for ways to offer information in a form that learners can accept, and even enjoy. Games have become a popular method to teach patients about health maintenance, disease prevention, or implementation of a treatment program.

Games allow students to test their knowledge in a nonthreatening situation. They require the learner to think about an issue or problem and apply new knowledge before using it independently. By providing a new twist to learning, games help patients learn, while they enjoy themselves and interact with others.

Immediate feedback is provided to the learner through scoring and discussion among the participants. In fact, a lively interaction between players usually ensues; this can spark a patient's interest and affect motivation positively (Crancer, 1981).

There are also disadvantages to using a game. As participants are selected, the nurse should keep in mind those factors that make gaming undesirable. Some people simply do not like games. Other patients may find it difficult to concentrate or understand the rules. When players focus entirely on accumulating points rather than on the subject matter presented in the game, very little learning takes place. Participants also need to set aside time to play the game. Finally, some players do not respond well to competition in that they become so upset if they are losing that they cannot participate in the discussion during and after the game. Playing a game in groups may decrease the threat of competition.

A game called "To Tell the Truth" is described by Hisgen (1981). Three contestants claim to be experts on a certain subject, in this case arthritis. Five panelists are given 2 minutes each to question the contestants from a question list about arthritis. The panelists make their decision as to who the real expert is and present the reasons for their choices. The expert stands up.

Mackey (1983) describes a picture charade game that is played like real charades except that instead of acting out words, participants are divided into groups and draw a picture of the word or phrase. In addition to drawing a picture, lines to indicate number of words or phrase may be drawn.

For instance, after using the newborn teaching plan, you decide to ask the parents to use their knowledge by playing picture charades with a list of ways to prevent children from ingesting poisons or foreign objects. The following phrases might be used:

- Never leave small objects within the child's reach.
- Always check all toys for safety (no loose small objects).
- Always keep medicine and poisons out of reach and locked up.
- Remember that babies are oral; everything goes into the mouth.
- Always keep ipecac in the medical closet; ask the physician for instruction.

It is relatively easy to develop your own game. Think of games that you played as a child and adapt them to what you want to teach. You can even change the rules and adjust the content of your game. The teaching plans in this book provide you with most of the information that you and your patient need to devise and play many games. For instance, the hypertension teaching plan will become the base for a hypertension game; the angina teaching plan, or the fractured hip teaching plan, can be used for other games.

When you develop a game, you should consider the same kind of criteria that you consider with other teaching techniques. The game should be constructed with a purpose and objectives. The format should be fully developed with guidelines or rules to govern play and should be fully tested. Finally, after every game is played, a 15- to 20-minute debriefing session should be scheduled to discuss why certain answers were correct or incorrect, where the participants had the most problems, and the subsequent action that should be taken to respond to the knowledge deficits that were highlighted in playing the game (Walljasper, 1982).

I adapted two games: a card sort game to teach medication and a quiz show game called "Breathing Easier" using the information found on the asthma teaching plan.

The card sort game can be played at a patient's bedside, using cards the size of playing cards. It is designed to allow a patient to use his knowledge of medication after completing the medication teaching plan. The objective of the game is to sort a group of cards into two stacks that indicate the name, action, dosage administration schedule, and side effects of the medication. The game can be adjusted in difficulty by adding or deleting elements of the card sort. For example, the first time the patient is asked only to sort cards indicating name of the drug, action, and time it is to be taken. Later, more cards representing dosage and side effects are added (Figure 4–1).

The game instructions follow:

- Essential information about the medication is reviewed with the patient.
- The patient is given a set of cards to sort into designated stacks.
- The nurse reviews the stacks and discusses the outcome of the game.
- The patient and the nurse then decide the need for further teaching.

The "Breathing Easier" game (Exhibits 4–6 and 4–7) can be played with two or three participants or by two groups. Groups may be less threatening and therefore more appealing to patients. The following rules of play are designated:

- A die is thrown or coin tossed to determine which group goes first.
- The group chooses a category of questions that it wishes to try to answer, in this case, diagnosis of asthma, administration of medication, special treatments, or follow-up of the problem.
- Questions are posed to the group starting with the least difficult (10-point questions) to the most difficult (60-point questions).

Figure 4–1 Card Sort Game

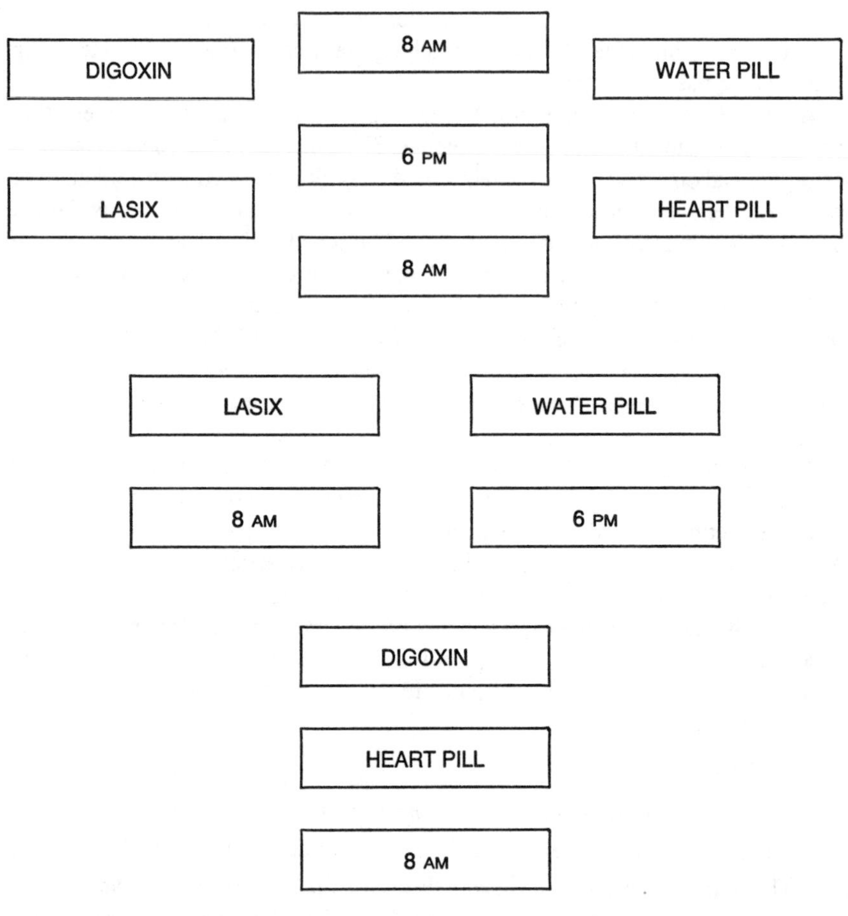

- When a question is missed, the next group chooses a category, and so on.
- The group accumulating the most points after all the categories are completed wins.

Role Playing

Role playing is a brief interaction in which individuals act out a scene and assume roles of people in that scene. In other words it is an animated case study, for instead of discussing the case, it is acted out. In a role play, individuals may play themselves or other people.

Exhibit 4–6 Breathing Easier: An Asthma Teaching Game

Diagnosis of Asthma	Administration of Medication	Special Treatment	Follow-up of Problem
10 points	10 points	10 points	10 points
20 points	20 points	20 points	20 points
30 points	30 points	30 points	—
40 points	40 points	40 points	40 points
50 points	50 points	50 points	—
60 points	60 points	60 points	—

Exhibit 4–7 Breathing Easier: An Asthma Teaching Game

Points	Diagnosis of Asthma	Administration of Medication	Special Treatment	Follow-up of Problem
10 points	Give a simple definition of asthma.	Name the medication you use for asthma.	Name the health maintenance tasks.	When is your next appointment?
20 points	Describe the anatomy of the lungs.	When do you take your medication and in what dose?	What services are available to help at home?	How will you contact your doctor or emergency room?
30 points	Describe the function of the lungs.	How does your medication work?	How would you arrange for oxygen?	—
40 points	What are the causes of asthma?	What are the side effects of your medication?	Describe five ways to control your environment.	List four reasons to contact your physician.
50 points	What are the signs and symptoms of asthma?	Describe when and why you would use an inhaler.	Describe how to do breathing exercises.	—
60 points	What changes occur in the lungs of patients who have asthma?	Describe how you would use an inhaler.	Describe how to do postural drainage.	—

Role plays are used to practice new behaviors or to experience the consequences of a new situation or interaction. An adolescent may play himself, and a nurse may play a friend as the patient explains the disease to the friend. The patient gets a chance to practice in a safe environment. The nurse can also teach a patient how to respond in these situations by reversing the roles. The nurse plays the patient, and the patient may play the friend. The patient is able to act out how the friend will react, and the nurse can demonstrate how to respond.

Role playing is also useful to explore feelings or to help people understand another's role. To help patients understand the relationships of the health care team, a case conference may be acted out. The patient is asked to identify the responsibilities or concerns of the physician, nurse, social worker, and physical therapist.

Role plays assist patients to understand themselves and others better. As a teaching technique, role plays are useful as a break in a lecture or in a group discussion. Participants become more attentive as they focus on a problem well known to all of them. They are also excellent tools to stimulate discussion and problem solving. After viewing a role play, the following questions might be asked: What was wrong with the scene? What was right? Was the problem clearly identified? If we were to act it out again, how would we change it? Through this type of discussion, issues are highlighted, and the nurse can ensure that the problem is clearly understood.

Case Method

Case method or case problem is a teaching strategy that utilizes a description of an account of a situation that a patient might encounter in real life. It may describe successful or unsuccessful problem solving. Patients are asked to put themselves in the situation, evaluate its cause, determine the consequences, and decide on appropriate action (Cooper, 1981).

Through case methods the learners apply the information that they have learned to real-life situations. In this setting, patients can step back and take their time to make a decision in a safe environment where they can clarify misconceptions and receive reinforcement for correct responses. For instance, many people may attribute a cause to a problem that is totally unrelated to the problem. Patients with congestive heart failure may attribute swollen ankles to standing on their feet all day and decide to sit down more often. How the patient perceives the cause will determine the treatment chosen. If the real cause of this patient's swollen ankles is that medication was not taken, sitting down more frequently may not relieve the swelling.

Through the presentation of real-life situations, patients can deal with concrete events and evaluate their ability to cope with these events. Case problems are an excellent method to make the patient aware that there is more information needed in order to handle problems comfortably at home.

For instance, after reviewing the hyper- and hypoglycemia teaching plan, the patient is given the following situation: "You have had a very busy week. You got 5 hours sleep last night. As you run out of the house, you realized that you hadn't had time to eat your usual breakfast. You had a quick lunch and met your mother at school. Suddenly you become weak, nauseated, and sweaty." The nurse then explores these questions: What is happening? How can you treat it? Why did it happen? How can you prevent it?

Case problems are also a good technique to evaluate how well patients apply knowledge acquired in other teaching plans. For example, after using the angina teaching plan, the following situation is described to a patient: "You are shopping in a downtown department store. As you are walking through the kitchen department, you feel a sharp heavy pressure in your chest, which radiates to your arm." What is the cause of the pain? What will make it better? What should you do if the pain persists?

Through these and other case problems both the teacher and learner can evaluate learning and identify areas that need reinforcement.

Demonstration and Return Demonstration

Demonstration is a teaching technique that may be used to show a patient how to perform a task step by step. The technique of demonstration is commonly used to teach a new skill such as to test for sugar and acetone or change a colostomy bag. It is also useful to show a patient that the task can be done.

Demonstration is also a way to show the results of certain actions or to explain cause and effect. The nurse may show a patient the result if an ace bandage is applied incorrectly or is the cause of a perfusion alarm going off.

It is very important that the demonstration is well planned and that the verbal and demonstration sequence is practiced to ensure that the patient views an organized, accurate presentation. If steps are deleted or actions are incorrect, the patient will be confused and left with many questions. The following points should be reviewed before every demonstration in order to help ensure success (Narrow, 1979):

- The expectations of the patient following the demonstration should be carefully outlined.
- Everyone must be able to see the demonstration clearly.
- The steps involved in successfully completing the task should be clearly defined and separated.
- The equipment used should be the same as the patient will use at home.

- Enough time should be allowed to run through the demonstration quickly to give the learners an idea of the task and to demonstrate the task slowly at least two more times.
- Printed material should be available to reinforce instruction.
- An appointment for everyone to practice the skill should be provided.

Return demonstration allows the learner to apply new knowledge and to receive feedback immediately. As the patient goes through the procedure that has been taught, reinforcement is given for correct performance and changes can be made if the task is done incorrectly.

Group Discussion

Group teaching is useful to encourage patients to express their feelings or share concerns with someone who has similar issues. Groups also allow people to learn from each other as they share experiences and explore meanings with others. Finally, group discussion is an efficient, economical way to teach several patients who have similar learning needs.

During group discussions new information is explored, reacted to, and applied in a personal way to each person in the group. Learning becomes individual as the experiences, attitudes, and reactions of others are seen in light of the patient's own situation; learning becomes very real (Narrow, 1979).

Patients who are going to surgery are commonly taught in a group. Other groups may include adolescent diabetics, pregnant teenagers, patients with a chronic disease such as hypertension or asthma, and people who are interested in the same health problem such as overeating or smoking cessation. Krumm, Vannata, and Sanders (1979) describe a group for teaching patients about chemotherapy.

As you develop your group, several factors need to be considered. First, you must select appropriate participants for the group. People with very high anxiety levels or painful experiences may be better taught, at least initially, outside the group, where more attention may be given to their personal needs.

Before the group is convened, consider the environment. Is the room comfortable? Can everyone see each other? Participation is enhanced if participants sit in a circle, around a table, or on comfortable chairs or sofas facing one another. Perhaps you would like to serve coffee, tea, or soda.

Begin the group by ensuring that everyone knows each other. Name tags can serve as a means of identifying each member. To help the members get to know one another, the nurse might ask each member to give some personal background and describe what the person wishes to get out of the group.

As you begin discussion, clarify the goals of the group. If the group is to meet more than once, discuss the long-term goals as well as the objectives for each session. You might then ask if the members find these goals acceptable, or wish to add goals or change the order of discussion. The participants can be asked to discuss the goals before the initial discussion begins or at the end of the meeting.

The group leader's role is to facilitate discussion, clarify misconceptions, provide information, and guide the group toward achievement of their goals. The nurse may begin by giving background information about the general focus of the group. For instance, for those patients going to surgery a description of pre-operative events is discussed. The nurse may help the group to share their experiences, offer empathy, and help them seek clarification and validation from each other. Participation should be encouraged without singling out a specific person who may want to remain silent. At times the nurse may need to refocus or direct discussion to meet the goals of the group. Most importantly the nurse should not lecture or monopolize the group but learn to listen, to tolerate moments of silence until members of the group feel comfortable sharing their thoughts and feelings (Redman, 1980; Narrow, 1979).

At the end of each session, the outcomes of the group should be evaluated. Ask the members what was learned. If the group is meeting only once, some members may wish to explore aspects of the discussion more fully. If so, provide an opportunity for further clarification later. If the group is to meet again, clarify the goals for the next session.

Self-Monitoring

Self-monitoring is a process in which individuals are actively involved in observing an undesirable health behavior that they wish to change (or is in the change process). In order for patients to control their behavior or responses, it is often beneficial for them to gain an acute awareness of their own behavior by carefully observing it. Monitoring can be used as a strategy that precedes a behavior change, or it can be used to reduce unhealthy activities without the individual consciously setting a goal for reduction. Awareness of the habit is sometimes stimulus enough for change (King, 1982).

Diaries or personal records are an effective means of self-monitoring (Baile & Engle, 1978). Patients may know that they drink too much or eat too much, but many do not realize the extent of their overindulgence until they keep careful track of each calorie, cigarette, or drink. Patients also are asked to observe not only specific health habits but also when these habits occur. They are asked to record the time of day (evening, morning), what they were doing (working, watching TV, talking with friends), and how they were feeling (happy, frustrated, or angry).

Obviously these methods are useful if learners take the time to become introspective and write down their observations. Glanz and Kirscht (1981) report the use of self-monitoring to increase the motivation of hypertensives to adhere to a drug regimen and to help patients adhere to weight loss recommendations.

This technique might also be very useful for cessation of smoking, reduction of alcohol consumption, reduction of asthmatic attacks, reduction of hypoglycemia episodes, or control of those habits contributing to constipation.

REFERENCES

Baile, W., & Engle, B. (1978). A behavioral strategy for promoting treatment compliance following myocardial infarction. *Psychosomatic Medicine 40*(5), 413–419.

Byrne, M., & Thompson, L. (1978). *Key concepts for the study and practice of nursing*. St. Louis: C.V. Mosby Co.

Cooper, S. (1981). Methods of teaching—revisited case method. *Journal of Continuing Education in Nursing 12*(5), 32–33.

Crancer, J., & Maury-Hess, S. (1981). Games: An alternative to pedagogical instruction. *Journal of Nursing Education 19*(3), 45–51.

Espich, J., & Williams, B. (1967). *Developing programmed instructional materials: A handbook for program writers*. Palo Alto, CA: Fearon Publishers.

Fisher, R., & Ury, W. (1981). *Getting to yes*. Boston: Houghton Mifflin Co.

Glanz, K., & Kirscht, J. (1981). Initial knowledge and attitudes as predictors of intervention effects: The individual management plan. *Patient Counselling and Health Education 3*(1), 30–41.

Hisgen, J.W. (1981). To tell the truth: A classroom gaming procedure. *Health Education 12*(1), 32–33.

Hughes, G. (1980). Manipulation: A negative element in care. *Journal of Advanced Nursing 5*(1), 21–29.

King, K. (1982). Selected behavioral strategies for the health educator. *Health Education 13*(3), 35–37.

Krumm, S., Vannata, P., & Sanders, J. (1979). Group approaches for cancer patients, a group for teaching chemotherapy. *American Journal of Nursing 79*(5), 916.

Lum, J.L., Chase, M., Cole, S., Johnson, A., Johnson, J.A., & Link, M.R. (1978). Nursing care of oncology patients receiving chemotherapy. *Nursing Research 27*(6), 340–346.

Mackey, R. (1983). Picture charades: A health teaching device. *Health Education 14*(7), 45.

Narrow, B. (1979). *Patient teaching in nursing practice: A patient and family centered approach*. New York: John Wiley & Sons, Inc.

Pool, J.J. (1980). Expected and actual knowledge of hospital patients. *Patient Counselling and Health Education 2*(3).

Redman, B.K. (1980). *The process of patient teaching in nursing*. St. Louis: C.V. Mosby Co.

Steckel, S.B. (1980). Contracting with patient-selected reinforcers. *American Journal of Nursing 80*(9), 1596–1599.

Steckel, S.B. (1982). *Patient contracting*. Norwalk, CT: Appleton-Century-Crofts.

Walljasper, D. (1982). Games with goals. *Nurse Educator 7*(1), 15–18.

SUGGESTED READINGS

Clark, M.C., & Bayley, E.W. (1972). Evaluation of the use of programmed instruction for parents maintained on warfarin therapy. *American Journal of Public Health 62*(8), 1135–1139.

Corbin, P.E. (1980). Health games, simulations and activities. *Health Education 11*(4), 24–25.

Herji, P.A. (1983). Hows and whys of patient contracting. *Nurse Educator 8*(1), 30–34.

McCormick, R.D., & Gilson-Parkevich, T. (1979). *Patient and family education tools techniques and theory*. New York: John Wiley & Sons, Inc.

Meyer, M.E. (1983). The puzzle design activity. *Health Education 14*(4), 41–42.

Petrillo, M., & Sanger, S. (1972). *Emotional care of hospitalized children*. Philadelphia: J.B. Lippincott Co.

Rankin, S.H., & Duffy, K.L. (1983). *Patient education: Issues, principles and guidelines*. Philadelphia: J.B. Lippincott Co.

Sloan, M.R., & Schommer, B.T. (1982). Want to get your patient involved in his care? Use a contract. *Nursing 82 12*(12), 48–49.

Steckel, S.B., & Swain, M.A. (1977). Contracting with patients to improve compliance. *Hospital 51*, 81–84.

Strecker, V.J. (1983). Improving physician-patient interactions: A review. *Patient Counselling and Health Education 4*(3), 129–135.

Taylor, P. (1982). Patient teaching: Keys to more success more often. *Nursing Life 2*(6), 25–32.

Zander, K., Bower, K., Foster, S., Towson, M., Wermuth, M., & Woldum, K. (1978). *A practical manual for patient teaching*. St. Louis: C.V. Mosby Co.

Zangari, M.E., & Duffy, P. (1980). Contracting with patients in day-to-day practice. *American Journal of Nursing 80*(3), 451–454.

Chapter 5

Developing Educational Tools

Virginia Ryan-Morrell and Karyl M. Woldum

WRITING A TEACHING PLAN

A teaching plan provides an organized, efficient tool to aid both the patient and the nurse as they pursue educational goals. In writing a teaching plan, the nurse must first consider what information the patient needs in order to return to a maximal state of health. For some teaching needs, the amount of information is too great to be contained in one teaching plan, for example, diabetes. In this case the information could be included in several different teaching plans: an insulin teaching plan, a urine testing teaching plan, and a diabetic foot care teaching plan. Once it has been established that one or several teaching plans are needed, the actual writing may be initiated.

A teaching plan has four sections:

1. purpose
2. content outline
3. learner objectives
4. evaluation

Each of these sections is addressed separately. The purpose, content outline, and learner objectives are contained in the body of the teaching plan. Optional guidelines are written in narrative form and printed separately.

The Purpose

The purpose includes one or more statements that describe the reason teaching is necessary. Common statements of purpose follow:

- To foster compliance with the treatment regime
- To lessen anxiety

- To promote self-care
- To assist the patient in understanding the disease and treatment

An example of a statement of purpose from the myocardial infarction teaching plan is "to assist the patient and family in understanding the pathophysiology of coronary artery disease."

Content

An outline of the subject matter contained in the teaching plan is described in the content. It helps to organize the information that is being given and ensures that every aspect of the teaching plan is addressed to the patient.

Learner Objectives

The content just discussed would be ineffective without the learner objectives described in the plan. All learner objectives should be written in behavioral terms. A behavioral objective identifies the behavior or behaviors that will be accepted as evidence that the learner has achieved an objective. It describes what a patient will be doing when demonstrating achievements and how a nurse can recognize this behavior. In other words, a behavioral objective defines an action (what the learner will be doing), defines the important condition under which the action will take place, and defines the quality of the action. For example, after receiving a description of the methods used to prevent urinary tract infections (important conditions), the patient demonstrates knowledge of prevention by naming (defines an action) three health habits (quality of action) that will reduce the chance of reinfection (Mager, 1975).

By using behavioral objectives, nurses can better evaluate teaching success and provide consistent direction for instruction. That is, they can clearly understand the subject matter and teaching method and materials to be used during instruction. Specific behavioral objectives also give learners a better comprehension of their goal in the learning process. Nurses' usual approach to teaching is to establish behavior patterns that are beneficial to a patient's health rather than to impart abstract theories. Many teachers never see the application of their teaching. Nurses will be able to see it and evaluate its effectiveness as their instructional sessions proceed. To aid in evaluation, the objective should clearly communicate your intent: "The best statement is the one that excludes the greatest number of possible alternatives to the goal" (Mager, 1975, p. 12). Avoid words that are open to many interpretations, e.g., *to know, to understand*. Instead, use words that describe precise behavior, something that can be measured, such as *describe, identify, list, demonstrate,* or *design*. Because the teaching plans define conditions under which our patients are taught (i.e., content and guidelines describe methodologies of teaching), it is not required that the condition be defined in every behavioral objective. An example of an acceptable objective would be "1. Given a list of foods, the patient identifies those which have a high potassium content." To ensure that each nurse teacher uses the same terminology in each successive teaching session, a more specific objective might be used: "1. Given a list of foods, the patient identifies oranges, bananas, and tomatoes as those with a high potassium content."

Evaluation

Upon completion of the teaching process or discharge from the hospital, an evaluation of the effectiveness of teaching should be documented. This section should describe the pace and complexity of the educational process. Was the learner capable of comprehending complex ideas or only the basics? What type of teaching strategies were effective? Finally, what is the plan for follow-up if the patient was unable to meet the essential objectives?

A teaching plan is a useful, efficient patient education tool. It provides a handy reference for the nurse and ensures a consistent approach to teaching throughout an illness or hospitalization. Teaching plans also decrease the time spent in writing lengthy progress notes. The plans in this book are intended as guides for other nurses who wish to develop additional tools for their patient.

WRITING A HANDOUT

Writing a patient handout offers the nurse yet another opportunity to utilize a variety of skills. After teaching the patient the appropriate information from the teaching plan, the nurse must then incorporate that information into an effective take-home tool for the patient. What is unique about writing a handout is that it presents the nurse with a chance to use skills that may be used in no other sphere of nursing.

Mrs. Green was a bright, motivated mother who was doing quite well mastering the technique of injecting her 6-month-old daughter Amy with Adrenocorticotropic hormone (ACTH). Mrs. Green was attentive during the teaching sessions and asked appropriate questions. When Mrs. Green and Amy were ready for discharge, the primary nurse gave Mrs. Green the telephone number of the unit with the instructions to call if she had any questions at all regarding the medication and its administration. Approximately 6 hours after discharge, the nurse was surprised to receive a phone call from Mrs. Green: "I know I've only been home a short time, but suddenly I feel very uncertain and confused about the baby's medicine. It's so different now that I'm home."

Mrs. Green offers the nurse an example of one of the most important reasons for writing and using patient handouts: to give the patient or significant other a *written account* of the treatment plan that they will be following at home. A handout allows the discharged patient to refer to important information taught during the hospitalization, in the changed environment—the home. Even the most successful hospital learner may falter when the supports of the hospital are no longer available. A well-written handout will reinforce previously discussed information and frequently give the patient the reassurance of a double-check while at home.

Writing a handout brings with it a certain responsibility. Whatever style of handout written, the nurse must be certain that the handout offers accurate information, is written in a manner that is understandable to the patient, and contains only information that has been previously introduced in teaching sessions.

It makes sense for the nurse to write the patient handout when writing the teaching plan. Since the nurse can utilize information from the teaching plan in the handout, it is wise to write the handout while the teaching plan information is still fresh.

The format or style of the handout may depend somewhat on the type and amount of information that must be covered. One format that is effective and quite popular is the question-and-answer style. A question is posed and then answered as clearly and thoroughly as possible. It is important when writing this type of handout that the nurse goes from the very general question gradually to the more specific. An example of this technique is seen in the handout that accompanies the gastric and duodenal ulcer teaching plan (Exhibit 5–1).

This handout answers common questions regarding ulcers while giving the patient valuable information about the disease. As seen by the example, the writer went from a general question (What is an ulcer?) to more specific areas (What are antacids and their importance in ulcer disease?). Questions progress in an orderly related fashion ("What is an ulcer?'' to ''What causes an ulcer?").

Another format of handout is one that describes in steps a technique that the patient has been asked to master. Obviously this style is appropriate for only certain subjects. However, if the patient has had to learn any information in a procedural step manner, this format is most effective.

Exhibit 5–1 Handout on Gastric and Duodenal Ulcer Teaching Plan

What is an ulcer?
What causes an ulcer?
What are the usual symptoms of an ulcer?
What is the standard treatment of an ulcer?
What are antacids and their importance in ulcer disease?
What symptoms should a physician be notified of?
What is the outlook for the patient who has an ulcer?

An example of this style can be seen in the handout accompanying the infant gavage feeding teaching plan (Exhibit 5–2).

It is helpful when writing this style of handout to divide steps into main categories such as inserting the feeding tube, gavage feeding, storage of equipment. Steps should be written in an organized, progressive manner.

One other format that may be used when writing a handout is the narrative format. This tends to be helpful when giving only small amounts of information. Since this is not often the case in patient teaching, this format is infrequently used.

Ideas to keep in mind while preparing your handout include the following:

- Choose words that are easily understood. Use simple sentence structure and avoid long complicated sentences that may be misleading or confusing. Keep

Exhibit 5–2 Handout for Infant Gavage Feeding

Inserting the Feeding Tube

1. Assemble necessary equipment.
2. Warm formula to room temperature.
3. Moisten and inspect mouth.
4. Measure feeding tube. Oral: measure from the tip of the nose to the mid-ear to the tips of the breastbone.
5. Tape tube securely.
6. Check for placement of the tube.
   a. Listen for a "pop" of air. Withdraw air.
   b. Remove residual from stomach, noting appearance and amount; replace residual.

Gavage Feeding

1. Flush formula through gavage set and attach to the feeding tube.
2. Offer pacifier if baby is able to suck.
3. Rate of flow is 2 to 4 ml/minute.
4. If infant gags or becomes restless, pinch tubing and wait until infant settles down.
5. If infant vomits, pinch tube and remove.
6. Call the pediatrician if any of the following occurs:
   a. bloody or green-tinged residual
   b. residual consistently more than half the previous feeding
   c. candidiasis (white patches inside the mouth)

Storage of Equipment

1. Reuse feeding tube and gavage set three or four times or until mild curds cannot be removed from the tubing.
2. Rinse the tubing and syringe with warm water after feeding.
3. Flush feeding tube with air, using the syringe, until water is removed from tubing.
4. Wrap feeding tube, gavage set, and syringe in a clean towel until the next feeding.

in mind that studies have shown that handouts written for an eighth-grade reading level are sometimes too difficult for a large percentage of the hospital population (Redman, 1972).

- Using illustrations is sometimes the most effective method of explaining a handout. Illustrations should be clearly and accurately drawn. They should be only as complicated as necessary.

Proper terminology should be used when labeling parts of the diagram. All of these terms, however, should be familiar to the patient before using the handout.

When illustrating body organs, provide the patient with a reference as to the size of the organ. (One patient believed that kidneys were not only bean-shaped but also bean-sized.)

Information contained in the handout is similar to that contained in the teaching plans. Therefore, if nurses wish to develop a handout for their patients, the teaching plans in this book are a convenient source of information. The nurse must remember, however, that a handout is intended only to be a reinforcement and reference for what has already been taught. A patient should not receive new information in a handout that has not been discussed during teaching sessions.

LINKING TEACHING PLANS WITH CARE PLANS

Standard care plans, like teaching plans, are a means of establishing a framework for nursing practice, for they identify the standards on which nurses measure the effectiveness of their care. In addition, new staff find them useful as a guide to routine care for patients with diagnoses that are unfamiliar to them. Standard care plans also decrease the time spent writing routine care and allow the nurse to be more creative in developing goals and interventions for patient's individual needs. For instance, nurses can spend an inordinate amount of time documenting the goals and interventions of a patient with diabetes. Through the use of standard care plans, the nurse can devote more time and energy to the patient's special needs.

The standard care plans used at the New England Medical Center outline the nursing diagnosis commonly associated with the patient's problem, the long- and short-term goals, and the appropriate nursing intervention to assist the patient achieve the goals. Included in every care plan is usually at least one nursing diagnosis of knowledge deficit or self-care deficit. When one of these diagnoses is identified, the goal is to meet the objectives of the appropriate teaching plan, and the nursing intervention is to review the teaching plan with the patient. In this way, teaching plans supplement the standard care plan, they do not duplicate the work.

For our purposes at our institution, goals and interventions for nursing diagnosis not related to teaching are developed and outlined on care plans (Exhibits 5–3, 5–4, and 5–5). Learning needs are identified on care plans, but the goals and interventions are developed on teaching plans (Appendix 5–A).

Exhibit 5–3 Myocardial Infarction Care Plan*

NURSING INDEX—MYOCARDIAL INFARCTION

Patient & Family Profile

Primary Nurse:

Date of Onset	Problem/Need	Expected Outcome	Dead-line	Goal Met	Nursing Intervention	Nsg. Intv. Completed	Eval. Date
	Potential for chest pain	Patient will be free from chest pain.			1. Obtain EKG on admission and daily as ordered. 2. Compare EKG and note any changes, i.e., evolution of myocardial infarction, presence and resolution of ischemia. 3. Check enzymes as ordered. 4. Oxygen as ordered. 5. Bedrest. 6. Nitroglycerin as necessary as ordered.		
	Potential for alterations in hemodynamics due to myocardial infarction	Patient demonstrates adequate perfusion as evidenced by —absence of diaphoresis —warm skin temperature —blood pressure ______ —unlabored respirations Lung sounds will have minimal congestion.			1. Monitor blood pressure and heart rate. 2. Monitor fluid status: strict intake and output; check urine specific gravity every shift, daily weights. 3. Note presence or increase of dependent edema. 4. Note skin temperature and color. 5. Check peripheral pulses every 4°. 6. Monitor rate and quality of respirations. Note use of accessory muscles. Auscultate lungs with each vital signs check.		

*The Myocardial Infarction Care Plan was written by Jeri F. Ricci, RN, BSN.

Exhibit 5–3 continued

NURSING INDEX—MYOCARDIAL INFARCTION (continued)

Patient & Family Profile

Primary Nurse:

Date of Onset	Problem/Need	Expected Outcome	Dead-line	Goal Met	Nursing Intervention	Nsg. Intv. Completed	Eval. Date
					7. Obtain baseline arterial blood gases. 8. Provide low flow oxygen as ordered.		
	Potential for arrhythmias due to myocardial infarction	Patient's arrhythmias will be controlled.			1. Check monitor rhythm strip every 2°; note rate, rhythm, intervals, presence of ectopy. 2. Prophylactic lidocaine as ordered. 3. Monitor serum electrolytes as ordered. 4. Maintain patent intravenous line. 5. Maintain adequate oxygenation. 6. EKG with change in heart rate or rhythm.		
	Decreased mobility due to restricted activity	Patient will demonstrate correct use of incentive spirometer and footboard. Patient will maintain a regular bowel routine without straining. Patient's skin integrity will remain intact. Patient is discharged free from complications of stasis.			1. Position change every 2°; check pressure points. 2. Provide passive range of motion exercises. 3. Encourage footboard exercises. 4. Use of incentive spirometer every hour while awake. 5. Administer minidose of heparin as ordered. 6. Administer stool softeners and offer commode as ordered.		

Exhibit 5–3 continued

NURSING INDEX—MYOCARDIAL INFARCTION (continued)

Patient & Family Profile

Primary Nurse:

Date of Onset	Problem/Need	Expected Outcome	Dead-line	Goal Met	Nursing Intervention	Nsg. Intv. Completed	Eval. Date
	Anxiety due to change in body image and decreased tolerance for physical activity	Patient verbalizes feeling about diagnosis. Patient feels safe in hospital environment. Patient tolerates increases in activity without signs and symptoms of cardiac stress.			1. Encourage ventilation of fears, explain procedures and equipment. 2. Familiarize patient with environment, use introduction to CCU teaching plan. 3. Support adaptive coping mechanisms. 4. Maintain restful atmosphere. 5. Sedatives as necessary and at hour of sleep as ordered to promote normal sleep patterns. 6. Limit activity and stress in environment as possible. 7. Maintain complete bedrest (may use commode if ordered). 8. Plan activities of daily living to maximize rest periods. 9. Out of bed after 2–3 days as ordered; monitor response to increased activity, i.e., change in heart rate, blood pressure, respiratory rate, chest pain.		

Exhibit 5–3 continued

NURSING INDEX—MYOCARDIAL INFARCTION (continued)

Patient & Family Profile

Primary Nurse:

Date of Onset	Problem/Need	Expected Outcome	Dead-line	Goal Met	Nursing Intervention	Nsg. Intv. Completed	Eval. Date
	Knowledge deficit due to new myocardial infarction	Patient states in simple terms an understanding of cardiac disease, activity restrictions, diet, medications, and need for medical follow-up.			1. Begin teaching, as tolerated by patient, using myocardial infarction teaching plan. Include family whenever possible.		

Exhibit 5–4 Fractured Hip Care Plan*

NURSING INDEX—FRACTURED HIP

Patient & Family Profile

Primary Nurse:

Date of Onset	Problem/Need	Expected Outcome	Dead-line	Goal Met	Nursing Intervention	Nsg. Intv. Completed	Eval. Date
	Alteration in comfort due to pain of fractured hip	Patient achieves pain control with medication and traction as evidenced by ______ ______			1. Medicate as ordered and position for comfort. 2. Maintain bucks traction with balanced suspension as ordered. 3. Trapeze over bed.		
	Knowledge deficit regarding hip surgery	Patient completes fractured hip teaching plan.			1. Refer to teaching plans.		
	Alterations in comfort due to postoperative pain	Patient states expectation of postoperative pain. Patient states pain is tolerated.			1. Medicate and position patient as ordered by the physician. 2. Maintain balanced suspension and bucks as ordered.		
	Impairment of skin integrity due to operating room procedure	Patient incision remains clean and intact.			1. Maintain initial dressing integrity; monitor and record drainage of davol and dressing. 2. After initial dressing change by the physician, dry sterile dressing to incision line and check daily.		

*The Fractured Hip Care Plan was written by Donna Gibbons, RN.

Exhibit 5–4 continued

NURSING INDEX—FRACTURED HIP (continued)

Patient & Family Profile

Primary Nurse:

Date of Onset	Problem/Need	Expected Outcome	Dead-line	Goal Met	Nursing Intervention	Nsg. Intv. Completed	Eval. Date
					3. Notify the physician of redness, heat, hematoma, or drainage from the incision. 4. Check temperature; check circulation, sensation, and motion every 4° for 48°, **then** as ordered.		
	Impaired physical mobility of affected extremity	Patient is free of hazards of immobility.			1. Skin care every ________ 2. Air mattress as necessary. 3. Respiratory care, i.e., chest physical therapy, triflow, turn, cough, and deep breathe every ________. 4. TEDs to unaffected limb; anticoagulants as ordered. 5. Monitor and maintain bowel status daily. Give stool softeners and laxatives as ordered as necessary. 6. Maintain ordered level of activity. 7. Administer anticoagulants as ordered.		

Exhibit 5–4 continued

NURSING INDEX—FRACTURED HIP (continued)

Patient & Family Profile

Primary Nurse:

Date of Onset	Problem/Need	Expected Outcome	Dead-line	Goal Met	Nursing Intervention	Nsg. Intv. Completed	Eval. Date
	Knowledge deficit of home management due to hip surgery	Patient and family completes objectives of fractured hip teaching plan:			1. Review the fractured hip teaching plan.		

Exhibit 5–5 Angina Care Plan*

NURSING INDEX—ANGINA

Patient & Family Profile

Primary Nurse:

Date of Onset	Problem/Need	Expected Outcome	Dead-line	Goal Met	Nursing Intervention	Nsg. Intv. Completed	Eval. Date
	Angina due to coronary artery disease.	Patient immediately describes chest pain to staff.			1. Encourage patient to notify staff when pain occurs. 2. Stress that the sooner the patient informs the staff, the sooner the pain can be relieved. 3. Ask the patient to describe the chest pain episode: location, intensity (use a scale of 1–10, 1 = mild, 10 = severe), radiation and presence of associated symptoms (shortness of breath, nausea, vomiting, diaphoresis, numbness or weakness in arms, wrists, hands, severe apprehension or feeling of impending death). 4. Document patient's typical (stable) angina so staff can be familiar with it. The typical chest pain is ________		

*The Angina Care Plan was written by Angela Martin, RN, BSN.

Exhibit 5–5 continued

NURSING INDEX—ANGINA (continued)

Patient & Family Profile

Primary Nurse:

Date of Onset	Problem/Need	Expected Outcome	Dead-line	Goal Met	Nursing Intervention	Nsg. Intv. Completed	Eval. Date
		Patient has less chest pain as evidenced by the following: ____________ _____less often _____less severe on a scale of 1–10 _____patient able to function and satisfied with relief			1. Give all cardiac medications, especially nitrates, on time. 2. Assist patient in maintaining limited activity if ordered. 3. If chest pain occurs, A. have patient stop what doing; B. check blood pressure and heart rate; C. follow orders, i.e., nitroglycerin, EKG, oxygen; D. if no orders, call physician; E. check blood pressure and pulse 5 minutes after each nitroglycerin and notify physician if hypertension occurs; F. document number of episodes and frequency of chest pain, also activity at onset; and G. check with physician regarding use of prophylactic nitroglycerin before the following activities known to chest pain: ____________		

Exhibit 5–5 continued

NURSING INDEX—ANGINA (continued)

Patient & Family Profile

Primary Nurse:

Date of Onset	Problem/Need	Expected Outcome	Dead-line	Goal Met	Nursing Intervention	Nsg. Intv. Completed	Eval. Date
					4. Beware of constipation. See constipation teaching plan.		
	Knowledge deficit regarding how to manage angina at home	Patient and family complete objectives of angina teaching plan.			1. Review angina teaching plan.		

Standard care plans in conjunction with teaching plans outline a guide for nursing practice and provide a basis on which to evaluate the consistency in which nurses achieve the outcomes for which they accept accountability.

REFERENCES

Mager, R.F. (1975). *Preparing instructional objectives*. Belmont, CA: Fearon Publishers.

Redman, B.K. (1972). *The process of patient teaching in nursing*. St. Louis: C.V. Mosby Co.

SUGGESTED READINGS

Goldberg, S. (1980). Do it yourself: A guide to writing patient literature. *Nursing Administration Quarterly* 4(2), 30–33.

McCormick, R.D., & Gilson-Parkevich, T. (1979). *Patient and family education tools, techniques, and theory*. New York: John Wiley & Sons, Inc.

Tucker, S.M., Breeding, M.A., Canobbio, M.M., Jacquet, G.D., Paquette, E.H., Wells, M.E., & Wellmann, M.E. (1975). *Patient care standards*. St. Louis: C.V. Mosby Co.

Zander, K., Bower, K., Foster, S., Towson, M., Wermuth, M., & Woldum, K. (1978). *A practical manual for patient teaching*. St. Louis: C.V. Mosby Co.

Appendix 5–A
Sample Teaching Plans

	Content/ Reinforcement Delivered Date & RN	Learner Objectives Met Date & RN	Not Applicable
ANGINA* **Purpose** To give information to the patient and family about the causes of angina, recognition of the symptoms of angina, and steps to take to relieve symptoms. **Content** I. Anatomy and physiology of the heart II. Pathophysiology of angina III. Symptoms of angina IV. Risk factors related to angina V. Situations that may precipitate anginal episodes VI. Home treatment of an angina episode VII. Care of nitroglycerin prescription VIII. Reasons to contact physician IX. Follow-up			
Learner Objectives I. The patient describes in simple terms the anatomy and physiology of the heart muscle and blood vessels. A. The heart muscle is a strong hollow organ that acts as a pump. It pumps blood throughout the body and lungs.			

*The Angina Teaching Plan was written by Melissa Flon, RN, BSN.

	Content/ Reinforcement Delivered Date & RN	Learner Objectives Met Date & RN	Not Applicable
B. The coronary blood vessels surround the heart and feed the heart muscle with blood containing oxygen and nutrients. II. The patient states in simple terms the definition and causes of angina. A. Angina is the discomfort caused by a decrease in the amount of blood feeding the heart muscle. B. Angina is a signal that there is temporary poor circulation to the muscle. C. The cause of angina may either be a buildup of fatty substances (cholesterol) on the lining of the blood vessels that feed the heart, or a sudden spasm of the blood vessels causing a slowing or stoppage of blood supply or both. III. The patient states the most common symptoms of angina. A. Chest or arm discomfort (tightness, squeezing, aching) B. Indigestion C. Aching that is felt in the neck, jaw, throat, shoulder, or back D. Breathlessness, weakness, sweating, dizziness E. My own symptoms are __________ IV. The patient defines risk factors and describes own controllable and uncontrollable risk factors. A. Risk factors are habits or characteristics that increase the probability of developing a narrowing of the blood vessels that feed the heart muscle. B. The controllable factors are 1. Cigarette smoking 2. High blood pressure 3. Increased amount of fatty substance in blood 4. Stress or tension 5. Lack of exercise 6. Obesity			

	Content/ Reinforcement Delivered Date & RN	Learner Objectives Met Date & RN	Not Applicable
C. Uncontrollable factors are 1. Diabetes 2. Family history 3. Males and persons over the age of 50 D. Patient's risk factors Controllable __________ __________ __________ Uncontrollable __________ __________ __________			
V. The patient states the situations that may precipitate an anginal episode: A. Sudden outbursts of activity or emotion, since they place unusual demands on the heart and increase its consumption of oxygen B. Heavy lifting such as picking up children, grocery bags, suitcases C. Activities such as stair climbing, prolonged walking, and sexual activity may overexert the heart D. Extreme temperature changes such as being out in cold or hot weather or showering in extreme hot or cold water E. Constipation with accompanied straining, which causes an increase workload on the heart F. Patient's anginal attacks are precipitated by the following: __________ __________ __________			
VI. The patient states the home treatment of anginal episodes. A. When the anginal episode begins, stop what I am doing. B. Place nitroglycerin tablet under the tongue. Note the time. C. If discomfort is not relieved, take another tablet under the tongue 5 minutes after the first.			

	Content/ Reinforcement Delivered Date & RN	Learner Objectives Met Date & RN	Not Applicable
D. Up to three tablets may be used, each 5 minutes apart, for each anginal episode.			
E. If discomfort is unrelieved, go to the nearest emergency room.			
F. After the discomfort is relieved, resume usual activity.			
VII. The patient states the care of nitroglycerin prescription.			
A. Nitroglycerin must be refilled every 4 to 6 months once the prescription has been opened.			
B. If nitroglycerin is fresh, it will burn or tingle under the tongue.			
C. It must be kept cool and in a dark container.			
D. A supply of tablets must be kept with the patient at all times.			
VIII. The patient states reasons to contact the physician or go to the emergency room:			
A. An angina episode not relieved after taking nitroglycerin			
B. Angina episodes occurring at rest			
C. Increasing severity of angina episode			
D. Increasing frequency of angina episode			
IX. The patient describes follow-up. Clinic physician #: __________ Local physician #: __________ Emergency room #: __________			
Evaluation			
If patient and/or significant others are unable to complete some or all of this teaching plan, document evaluation in progress notes.			
MYOCARDIAL INFARCTION*			
Purpose			
To assist the patient and family in understanding the pathophysiology of coronary artery disease leading to a myocardial infarction. To assist the patient and family in identifying guidelines for home care related to myocardial infarction.			

*The Myocardial Infarction Teaching Plan was written by Patricia McLaughlin, RN, BSN, and Shelley MacDonald, RN, BSN.

	Content/ Reinforcement Delivered Date & RN	Learner Objectives Met Date & RN	Not Applicable
Content I. Anatomy and physiology of the heart muscle II. Anatomy and physiology of the heart's blood supply III. Atherosclerosis in the development of coronary artery disease IV. Angina V. Definition and symptoms of myocardial infarction VI. Risk factors related to individual life style VII. Home care of the myocardial infarction patient VIII. Reasons to contact physician IX. Follow-up			
Learner Objectives I. The patient describes the anatomy and physiology of the heart. A. The heart is a strong hollow muscle that pumps blood to all parts of the body and lungs. II. The patient describes the anatomy and physiology of the heart's blood vessels. A. Vessels that surround the heart to feed blood containing oxygen to the heart muscle are called *coronary arteries*. B. The coronary artery system has three major branches: the right main and circumflex coronary artery supplying blood to both the right and left side of the heart and the left coronary artery supplying blood to the left side of the heart. III. The patient describes the development of coronary artery disease from atherosclerosis. A. Fatty layers (plaque) form and accumulate on the lining of the coronary arteries. B. This plaque is usually made up of cholesterol, which can block the blood vessels and prevent them from delivering blood to the heart muscle.			

	Content/ Reinforcement Delivered Date & RN	Learner Objectives Met Date & RN	Not Applicable
IV. The patient meets the learner objectives of the angina teaching plan. V. The patient describes the physiology of myocardial infarction and the symptoms associated with it. A. A myocardial infarction is an injury to an area of the heart muscle caused by a blocked coronary artery. B. Soon after the myocardial infarction, the heart begins to heal through formation of scar tissue, which strengthens the damaged muscle. C. Symptoms of a myocardial infarction vary with each individual. Some of the most common symptoms are 1. Chest discomfort 2. Pain 3. Pressure that may extend to the neck, jaw, or arms 4. Nausea 5. Perspiration 6. Dizziness 7. Weakness 8. Apprehension D. Description of the patient's own symptoms: ____________________ VI. The patient describes a risk factor and states the controllable and uncontrollable risk factors of own life style. A. Risk factors are certain habits or characteristics that increase a person's chances of developing narrowing of the coronary arteries. B. Controllable factors 1. Smoking 2. High blood pressure 3. Increased amounts of fatty substances (cholesterol) in the blood 4. Stress or tension 5. Lack of exercise 6. Obesity C. Uncontrollable factors 1. Diabetes 2. Family history of coronary artery disease 3. Males and people over the age of 50			

	Content/ Reinforcement Delivered Date & RN	Learner Objectives Met Date & RN	Not Applicable
D. Patient's risk factors Controllable ________________ ________________ ________________ Uncontrollable ________________ ________________ ________________			
VII. The patient describes the guidelines for home care during the first 2 weeks after discharge as discussed with the primary nurse and physician. A. Activity 1. Walking ________________ 2. Stairs ________________ 3. Bathing ________________ 4. Travel in a car ________________ 5. Housework ________________ 6. Sexual Activities ________________ B. Medications. The patient completes the general medication teaching plan for each discharge medication. C. Diet. The patient describes diet restrictions as discussed with dietitian. ________________			
VIII. Reasons to call the physician A. Recurrence of symptoms that brought the patient to the hospital initially B. Side effects of medications taken at home C. Questions related to activities discussed in the hospital			
IX. Follow-up A. Next appointment: __________ B. Phone MD: __________ ER: __________ Clinic: __________			

	Content/ Reinforcement Delivered Date & RN	Learner Objectives Met Date & RN	Not Applicable
C. If appropriate, the patient and/or significant others complete the following teaching plans: 1. Angina 2. Hypertension 3. CHF 4. Cardiac catheterization 5. Medication			
Evaluation If patient and/or significant others are unable to complete some or all of this teaching plan, document evaluation in progress notes.			

GUIDELINES: HOME CARE FOR MYOCARDIAL INFARCTION PATIENT

To the Nurse

When designing an activity home care guide for your patient, please use the following information as a reference. You must discuss with the physician involved in the patient's care what this individual patient requires as a proper guide for activity. Plan together, using what the patient states as normal routine at home before this hospitalization. Remember that each patient is an individual, and the activity guide must be realistic to the person's life style.

Learner Objective VII

The patient describes the activity and diet guidelines for the first 2 weeks after discharge.

Walking

When walking at home, stay on level ground or the floor. Do not hurry. Go outside if the weather is mild. If the weather is too cold or too hot, it may cause your heart to work harder.

Stairs

When climbing stairs, go up slowly, stopping on each step to rest.

Bathing

When showering, avoid hot or very cold water, hurrying, or excessive scrubbing or drying off.

Travel in a Car

A family member may drive you to a level place for taking your short walks. You can usually take short trips (for example, to the grocery store). When carrying objects, they should weigh less than 5 pounds.

Housework

Light housework (for example, help prepare meals or wash dishes), remembering to keep arms at waist level.

Sexual Activities

Sexual relations with your usual partner requires about the energy to climb two flights of stairs. Many people participate in sex a month after their heart attack. Give yourselves plenty of time for sex and minimize the chances for interruptions by taking the phone off the hook and making sure that children are occupied.

If you are tired or have recently eaten a large meal, have sex later.

Be in a good mood.

Return to the usual positions unless you would just like to change or these positions seem strenuous to you.

If you are prone to angina, take a nitroglycerin before sex. If angina develops during intercourse, stop and rest.

PATIENT HANDOUT FOR HOME CARE

The patient describes the guidelines for home care during the first 2 weeks after discharge as discussed with the primary nurse and physician.

A. Activity

____

____

1. Walking

____

____

2. Stairs

____

____

3. Bathing

____

____

4. Travel in a car

____

____

5. Housework

____

____

6. Sexual activities

____

____

B. Diet restrictions—after discussion with dietitian.

____

____

C. Reasons to call the physician
   1. Recurrence of symptoms
   2. Side effects of medication
   3. Questions related to activities

Index

M

N

O

P